Steroids

Scott E. Lukas, Ph.D.

—The Drug Library—

ENSLOW PUBLISHERS, INC.

44 Fadem Road   P.O. Box 38
Box 699   Aldershot
Springfield, N.J. 07081   Hants GU12 6BP
U.S.A.   U.K.

Library of Congress Cataloging-In-Publication Data

Lukas, Scott E., Ph.D.
    Steroids / Scott Lukas
        p. cm. — (The Drug Library)
    Includes bibliographical references and index.
    ISBN 0-89490-471-X
    1. Doping in sports—Juvenile literature. 2. Anabolic steroids—
Health aspects—Juvenile literature.
    [1. Steroids. 2. Athletes—Drug Use. 3. Drug abuse.] I. Title. II. Series.
RC1230.L85 1994
362.29'088796—dc20   93-38524
                                                              CIP
                                                              AC

Printed in the United States of America.

10 9 8 7 6 5 4 3 2

Illustration Credits: Data are from M.H. Williams, *Beyond Training: How Athletes Enhance Performance Legally and Illegally*, (1989, Champaign, Il: Leisure Press.), p. 16; Dr. J. Keul, p. 100; Dr. Pope and Dr. Katz, 1988, American Journal of Psychiatry, 145, p. 55; Dr. Scott E. Lukas, pp. 26, 36, 46, 58, 67, 87, 97; Provided by Larry D. Bowers, Ph.D., Sports Medicine Drug Identification Laboratory, Indiana University Medical Center, Indianapolis, IN, p. 28; Reprinted with permission from C.R. Moore in *Sex and Internal Secretions*, 1939, Williams & Wilkins Publishing Co., p. 10.

Cover Photo: © The Stock Market/Lew Long 1993.

Contents

Introduction

Drug abuse is the most serious problem facing today's youth. Many doctors, scientists, lawmakers and police officers are concerned about drugs like alcohol, cocaine, marijuana, and tobacco. These are very addictive drugs that are abused by many adolescents and adults. But the use and abuse of steroids has increased recently, and today's youth do not know very much about these chemicals. Steroids are a group of natural and artificial chemicals called hormones that produce male-like effects in both males and females. It has been estimated that over one million Americans use steroids. There may be as many as five hundred thousand teenage users.

The main reason that so many people use steroids is that both amateur and professional athletic sports are very competitive and everyone wants to win—at any cost. Drugs have been used for centuries to improve performance. The ancient Greek Olympians used a strong stimulant, strychnine, and hallucinating mushrooms to get "psyched up" before the games.[1] In 1886, a French cyclist was the first athlete to die from a performance drug. He took a mixture of cocaine and heroin called speedballs. This is the same drug combination that killed John Belushi, the actor and comedian of the TV show *Saturday Night Live.*

Many athletes still train with long workouts, but others are taking steroid shortcuts to improve their performance. Steroids can increase muscle size and weight gain. It is not clear if they improve performance, but they do cause serious bad effects to the body and can increase aggressive behavior. The use of steroids to improve performance in sporting events is illegal, and all steroids are banned from athletic competition.

The second reason people take steroids is to look more attractive. Many people think they will be more popular if they have the "perfect" body. Steroids must be obtained through prescription for the various legal uses, but many users get them illegally. The most frequent places to get these black market steroids are health clubs and gyms and through mail order from Europe, Canada, and Mexico. Steroid use is legal in these countries. It is estimated that $100 million to $400 million is spent on illegal steroids each year.[2]

1

What Are Steroids?

The term steroid refers to a group of chemicals that are found in many plants and animals. Most steroids found in humans look a lot like cholesterol. Toad poisons and chemicals from the digitalis or foxglove plant are also steroids. The steroids found in plants are good insect repellents, and the toad steroids taste bad to other animals. Different glands in the human body make steroids, which act as hormones. A hormone is a chemical that helps body organs do their jobs. Certain hormones only work on specific organs. For example, insulin is a hormone that helps us use sugar for energy. Growth hormone helps our bones grow longer, and thyroid hormone helps us manage our energy supplies. The most familiar steroid hormones are testosterone, the natural male sex hormone, and estrogen, the natural female sex hormone. Birth control pills are made of types of estrogen and progesterone, another female steroid hormone.

Testosterone — The Male Hormone

Testosterone is made in the testes of males. A small amount is also made in the adrenal glands. Estrogen is made in the ovaries of females. However, a small amount of testosterone is also made in the ovaries of women.[1] Only the male hormone, testosterone, affects growth. Estrogen helps produce the typical female characteristics such as smooth skin, high-pitched voices, wider hips, and a distribution of fat that forms the breasts and hips. It is testosterone, and other steroids like it, that has caused such concern in sports medicine these days.

All cholesterol-like steroids have rings. Different steroids are made by changing the number and type of attachments of the rings.

Some people confuse the anabolic steroids with corticosteroids. The natural corticosteroids such as cortisol, corticosterone, and cortisone help our bodies use proteins and carbohydrates. Another steroid, aldosterone, helps regulate the amount of salt and water in our bodies. These steroids are made by the adrenal gland, which is located on top of our kidneys. Corticosteroids such as prednisone and hydrocortisone are often used to treat infections, arthritis (inflammation of the joints), asthma (difficulty in breathing), and certain types of cancers. These drugs do not build up muscle like testosterone. The male-like, androgenic effects of these chemicals are often combined with the tissue-building, anabolic effects. Since all male-like hormones have some amount of tissue-building action, the term anabolic-androgenic steroid is the preferred name for these chemicals. However, to make it easier to read this book, the word steroid will be used to mean only the anabolic-androgenic steroids like testosterone.

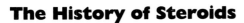

The History of Steroids

The history of how the male-like hormones were found is very interesting. Castration is a surgical procedure to remove the testes of a male animal. It has been known for many hundreds of years that castration of male animals prevents them from being able to make babies and to develop sexually. Castration has been used by farmers for many years. It helps domesticate, or tame, male livestock and improve the production of meat. Many years ago, choir boys were castrated by some churches. After castration, these boys kept their very high soprano voices for many years. Ancient civilizations also castrated certain men, creating special servants called eunuchs to guard the king's harems.[2] Before 1849, scientists thought that the changes in body size and shape, and the high-pitched voice that occur after castration were caused by the nervous system.

In the mid-1800s, a man by the name of Berthold did a series of experiments with roosters to find out why castration caused infertility (the inability to make babies) and a loss of the secondary sex characteristics (such as facial and body hair and a deeper voice).[3] When the rooster's testes were removed, the fleshy crest on its head (called the comb) became much smaller. However, if the testes were put back into the bird, the comb did not shrink at all. (The results of this experiment are shown on page ten. The bird on the left is a normal brown leghorn rooster with a well-developed comb. The bird on the right had his testes removed and has no comb.) Scientists thought that a substance produced by the testes must be moving through the blood to the rooster's comb. Other scientists later identified a chemical from the testes. When this chemical was

9

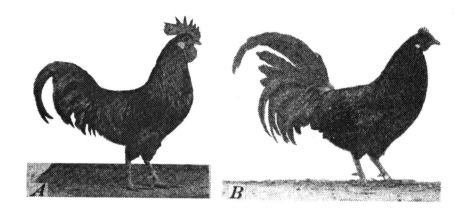

Figure 1.

The effects of removing the testes on the comb of the brown leghorn rooster are shown here. The rooster on the right shows no comb on the top of his head, after his testes are removed.

injected into a castrated male, it prevented the effects of castration.[4]

In the late 1800s, the well-respected French scientist, Dr. E. C. Brown-Sequard, made an amazing "discovery." He claimed to have found the cure for old age. He had injected portions from testicles into older animals and found that the effects of old age were reversed. He even tried some of the potion on himself. In his paper, he wrote the following:

> *I am seventy-two years old. My general strength, which has been considerable, has notably and gradually diminished during the last ten or twelve years. Before May 15th last, I was so weak that I was always compelled to sit down after a half an hour's work in the laboratory. Even when I remained seated all the time, or almost all the time, in the laboratory, I used to come out of it quite exhausted after three or four hours experimental labour, and sometimes after only two hours.[5]*

His report continued:

> *The day after the first subcutaneous injection, and still more after the two succeeding ones, a radical change took place in me, and I had ample reason to say and write that I had regained at least all the strength I possessed a good many years ago. Considerable laboratory work hardly tired me. To the great astonishment of my two principal assistants, Drs. D'Arsonval and Henocque, and other persons, I was able to make experiments for several hours while standing up, feeling no need whatever to sit down.*

His discovery was, unfortunately, not true. The results could not be duplicated. Dr. Brown-Sequard had not found a fountain of youth. Apparently, he was having a placebo response, or reacting to an imagined stimulus. However, his report stimulated many other scientists to study the interesting effects of a substance that was in the testicles. Since scientists still did not know what the chemical looked like, it was very hard to find it. A clue came in the early 1930s when German scientists tried to identify this chemical. They collected 25,000 liters of urine from male policemen. After many experiments, they finally ended up with fifteen milligrams of a chemical they called andosterone.[6,7] A few years later in 1935, scientists working in Amsterdam collected ten milligrams of a chemical from one hundred kilograms of bull testes.[8] This chemical was identified as testosterone.

There are a number of man-made or artificial steroids that have a chemical structure that is similar to testosterone. These artificial steroids are made by drug companies. Artificial steroids are needed because doctors cannot get enough of the real hormone from natural sources to treat certain diseases in people. Many of these steroids (both natural and artificial) are also used by veterinarians to treat medical problems in animals. In addition, farmers give steroids to their cattle to increase their size. This helps increase meat production. The artificial, or synthetic, steroid hormones differ mostly in how much you must take and the number of side effects they produce. A side effect is a reaction to a drug that is not wanted but happens anyway. Some steroids are given by injection, and others are swallowed as a pill. These two types have similar muscle-growing effects but have different side effects.

Questions For Discussion

1. Why do you think that both men and women have both kinds of sex hormones instead of just one?

2. What do you think would happen if a woman athlete who was pregnant with a female baby took testosterone during her pregnancy?

3. Dr. Brown-Sequard conducted an experiment on himself by taking the potion he had made. We now know that his reaction was due to the placebo effect. How could he have improved his experiment to avoid this error?

4. Do you think artificial steroids are more or less dangerous than the natural steroids produced in our bodies?

2

Who Uses Steroids?

In 1939, scientists suspected that the sex steroid hormones might improve physical or athletic performance. Scientific studies conducted in 1944 confirmed this first impression. It is rumored, but has never been proven, that one of the earliest uses of steroids was by Hitler's troops. It was thought that steroids would help increase their fighting ability.[1] After World War II was over, many prisoners were found in concentration camps. They were starving. The first medical use of steroids was to treat these prisoners who had not eaten for a long time. These drugs helped them build up their body weight again.

Steroid Use by Athletes

The first use of anabolic steroids in sports was by the Soviet weight-lifting teams in the early 1950s.[2] The Russian athletes took such high doses that the women began to look like men. In fact, sports organizations began to give chromosome tests to the women to make sure that they were, in fact, women. Soon thereafter, American strength athletes began using these drugs on a wide scale. Within a few years, the use of steroids became more common among athletes in endurance sports, such as long-distance marathon runners and swimmers.[3] Use by high school athletes was suspected as early as 1959.[4] Professional football players began using steroids soon thereafter. Use by nonathletes has been a very recent trend.[5] These people use them just to improve their appearance.

Until the mid-1970s, information such as who is using steroids and how much they are using was based solely on stories by individuals and rumors. Although many rumors are still widely believed, more accurate estimates of steroid use are now available. This is because a number of scientific surveys have now been conducted.[6,7,8,9,10]

Steroid use in other sports has also been studied. It is now known that weight lifters, power lifters, and bodybuilders are the primary users of steroids.[11] Over 50 percent of male and 10 percent of female bodybuilders report using steroids. Figure 2 shows the percentage of these and other athletes who use steroids. A very large percent of the male athletes in these sports have used or will use steroids. The percentages are slightly lower for other athletes, including those in field sports such as shot put and discus and football players. Only about 10 percent of the long-distance runners use steroids. Use by female athletes is much lower and ranges from 20 percent in strength sports participants to 12 percent in endurance runners. In 1990, a survey was conducted to determine how many professional football players used steroids. Over one thousand six hundred

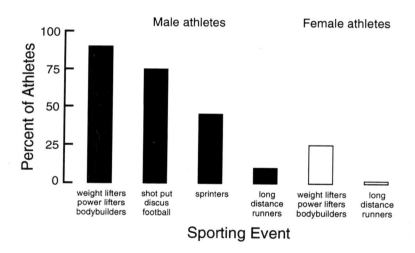

Figure 2

The percentage of different athletes who reportedly use steroids is shown here.

players were asked to complete the questions. Only 120 players filled out the questionnaires. About 28 percent of the players reported using steroids. However, 67 percent of the offensive linemen used steroids. A smaller percentage of the receivers and quarterbacks used them. One effect of steroids reported to be "beneficial" is the increase in aggression or hostile behavior. It is thought that the linemen use the steroids to help them get pumped up to combat their opponent.

Steroid Use by Adolescents

Currently, professional and amateur athletes are the main users of steroids, but use is increasing in the general population too. Use by professional athletes is a big problem, but use by adolescents is very disturbing. In 1971, a survey was conducted in Arizona. The scientists found that only 1 percent of high school students used steroids. The results of more recent surveys shows that the problem has grown. A variety of national surveys conducted since 1987 have found that 5 to 16 percent of male high school seniors now use, or have used, steroids at least once in their life.

The year 1988 was called the "Year of Steroids" because so many athletes were caught taking them at various sporting events, including the Olympics.

At the end of 1988, scientists from Pennsylvania State University published the results of a survey they conducted. They sampled 3,403 male high school students and found that 6.6 percent of male high school seniors use, or have used, steroids. This meant that as many as five hundred thousand male students across the United States had experience with steroids. Dr. Buckley and his colleagues were very surprised to find that over two-thirds of them started using these drugs before they turned sixteen years old. The reasons that the students used steroids were also very interesting. Almost half of them said they used steroids to help them play their sports. About 11 percent said that steroids helped them either to prevent an injury or helped them to heal. Almost one-third of the students said that they used steroids simply to improve their appearance. It was very surprising to find this many students using steroids who did not play any sports. About 30 percent of the students were using needles to inject the steroids. Female students do not seem to be using steroids as much as males. Only 1.3 percent of the female high school seniors reported using steroids.[12]

There is a very alarming trend of use among young people. Another survey conducted in 1989 found that 2 percent of sixth graders in Maryland used steroids.[13] A survey of 1,881 ninth graders was conducted by Dr. Robert Durant and his colleagues at the Medical College of Georgia.[14] They found that 5.4 percent of the males and 1.5 percent of the females were using steroids without a prescription. Of these steroid users, 25 percent reported sharing needles to inject the drugs. In addition, the males and females who used steroids were very likely to be using other drugs of abuse, including cocaine, alcohol, marijuana, tobacco cigarettes, and smokeless tobacco. It is a well-known fact that the HIV virus that causes Acquired Immunodeficiency Disease (AIDS) is transmitted by sharing needles. This is very disturbing behavior in such a young population and places these young people at risk for getting AIDS.

Another very disturbing finding comes from a survey that was completed in July 1993 by Vince Stigler.[15] Stigler is a graduate student at Indiana University and will be submitting his results for publication. He questioned 873 high school football players from twenty-seven different high schools across the state of Indiana. Over 6 percent of them used steroids. Stigler also asked them how old they were when they first started taking steroids. Fifteen percent were ten or younger and another 15 percent were between eleven and twelve years old. The largest percentage, 36 percent, started between the ages of thirteen and fifteen and 33 percent started between sixteen and eighteen years old. This is the first time that steroid use has been found in boys under the age of ten.

Steroid use by college students is also increasing. In 1970, 15 percent of college athletes used steroids. By 1984, 20 percent were using them.[16] About 9 percent of the football players and 4 percent of the track and field athletes used steroids. Also, these surveys found that 4 percent of basketball players, 3 percent of the baseball players and 4 percent of tennis players all used steroids. Use by female college athletes is much lower (about 1 percent). Reported users were in track and field sports (1 percent), basketball (1 percent) and swimming (1 percent).

Patterns of Steroid Use

The way in which steroids are used is very different from other drugs like cocaine, marijuana, or alcohol. These "typical" drugs of abuse are taken to feel good and to forget problems. They are taken for their immediate effects on the brain and body. Steroids do not affect the brain like other drugs of abuse and so do not produce a "high" or euphoria. Instead, the patterns of steroid use are chosen mainly to increase muscle growth.

Steroids are most often taken in a cycle. Each cycle lasts from four to eight weeks. Six weeks is the most common cycle length. The reason that steroids are taken this way is because they need time to change the body's chemistry and to produce more muscle. After six weeks, most users will then stop taking steroids for a few weeks or months. Many times, the reason that they stop is because they plan to compete in a sport and they do not want the steroids to be found in their urine. These cycles are then repeated. Sometimes, a heavy user can complete six or seven cycles per year.

Another practice that is done only with steroids is that users "stack" different drugs together. Some very experienced weight lifters will use as many as six different steroids at the same time. These users claim that these special mixes give them the right balance of desired effects. There is no scientific proof that stacking is better than using just one steroid at a time. It is interesting that many of the steroids used by bodybuilders are supposed to be used in animals, such as horses, cats, and dogs. These athletes do not seem to mind using a drug that is not approved for use in humans.

Questions For Discussion

1. What are some of the benefits to chromosome tests?

2. Why do you think that weight lifters, power lifters and bodybuilders are the primary abusers of steroids?

3. What do you think would happen to an eleven-year-old boy who starts to take high doses of testosterone in order to look good? How many more inches do you think he will grow in the next four to five years?

4. Why do you think an abuser "stacks" or mixes different steroids?

3

Are Steroids Legal?

Steroid use is not legal in sports today. It should be remembered that other drugs such as cocaine, marijuana, and alcohol also are not permitted. But steroids are very helpful in treating certain diseases. Before the legal issues of steroid use are discussed, it is important to know how these drugs are detected in a person's body. Every drug that is taken either by mouth or by injection is broken down by the liver and then eliminated from the body. When a drug is broken down, or metabolized, the remaining chemicals are called metabolites. One of the more common ways for a drug and its metabolites to be excreted is through the urine. Scientists can detect which drugs a person has taken simply by analyzing the person's urine.

Medical Uses for Steroids

Steroids can be very useful drugs when given by a doctor for a specific disease or problem.[1] For example, doctors give testosterone to men who cannot make enough of their own testosterone. These men have what is called androgen deficiency disease. Testosterone is also used to treat certain types of blood diseases like anemia and kidney failure. Anemia occurs when there are not enough red blood cells. Patients who have problems with muscle production or whose muscle is broken down can also be helped by steroids. For example, patients with certain forms of cancer, burns, and AIDS can be treated with steroid hormones. Also, steroids often can help a person who has had a major accident.

Sometimes, steroids are used to treat adolescent boys who have certain disorders. Some boys do not reach puberty until age fourteen or fifteen. These boys may have social problems because of their small size. Also, if the boy was very good at sports when he was eleven or twelve, he may no longer be able to compete with the bigger boys by age thirteen. This can be very frustrating to a developing boy. Doctors will sometimes treat these boys with a small dose of a testosterone-like drug for three months. In another disorder, the penis is too small for urination to occur. Steroid treatment can correct this problem too. Finally, some children fail to grow taller. Now, doctors can give steroids along with growth hormone to improve an adolescent's growth rate.

However, it is the nonmedical use of steroids by athletes and, more recently, by nonathletes that has increased attention and concern in recent years. The major reason for this concern is that steroids are very powerful drugs. The amount of drug that is taken by these athletes is often fifty to one hundred times the amount used by doctors to treat diseases. Like other drugs, too much of a steroid can lead to toxic effects and, in some cases, even death.

Urine Testing for Steroids

Today, urine testing is being done for international, national, and college programs. Now, even high school athletic programs and military and law enforcement agencies are testing for these drugs. Testing was first designed to catch athletes who are using steroids. However, urine tests are now being done during screening for jobs in the work place.

Steroids were first banned by the International Olympic Committee in 1975. The next year, in Montreal, Canada, the committee began to test the urine of athletes for steroids. Of the 275 urine samples taken, only 2.9 percent were positive. In 1986, the National Collegiate Athletic Association (NCAA) began to test football players who were in championship bowl games. Over the years, the number of athletes who were found to have taken steroids ranged between 0.1 and 2.0 percent. However, this low rate was found because the tests were announced beforehand. If an athlete knows when the test will be performed, then he or she can stop taking the steroids in time for the drug to get out of the body. A different result occurs when the tests are not announced. In 1984, the International Olympic Committee gave surprise urine tests at some Olympic sporting events. They found that about 50 percent of the athletes had taken steroids.[2]

The most publicized case of steroid abuse was at the 1988 Summer Olympic Games. Ben Johnson, the Canadian sprinter, had his gold medal taken away because a steroid was found in his urine. The steroid he took is called stanozolol. It is sad that no one remembers who really won that 100-meter race—it was Carl Lewis from the United States. He finished in 9.92 seconds, just

13/100 of a second behind Ben Johnson. Would a little bit more training without steroids have helped Ben Johnson win the medal legally and fairly? Ben Johnson was punished by not being allowed to run in international races for two years. He probably lost millions of dollars in fees for appearing places and for endorsing certain products.[3]

Drugs were a big problem in the 1988 Olympic games. Two Bulgarian weight lifters, Mitko Grablev and Angel Guenchev, had their gold medals taken away because they were taking a drug that increases urine production.[4] This drug is often used to hide steroid use. Even though the Bulgarian team still had five events left, the whole team withdrew from the games after their teammates were caught.

Measuring Steroids in the Body

A special machine called a gas chromatograph (GC) is used to measure steroids in the urine. This machine is very accurate, and it can measure thousands of different chemicals. The illustration on page twenty-six shows what a GC looks like. The samples of urine are processed in the circular bin located on the left. Small amounts of the urine are sprayed onto a column that helps separate the various chemicals. The sample then goes into an oven, and the amount of each chemical is measured. An example of a GC report is shown on page twenty-eight. This one is positive for steroids.

However, there are still some problems with the GC procedure. The biggest problem is that the amount of drug being measured in the body is very small. Also, since the body normally makes testosterone, it is hard to prove that a person is injecting extra testosterone into his or her body. The only method for detecting illegal testosterone is to measure the proportion of

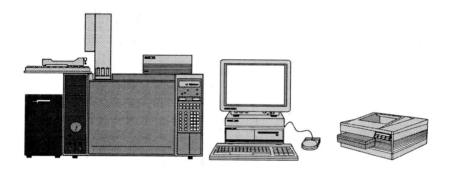

A gas chromatographic instrument used to detect and measure the amount of steroids in blood or urine specimens is shown here.

testosterone to its metabolite, epitestosterone.[5] Normally, the amounts of testosterone and epitestosterone are the same. If a person has six times as much testosterone as epitestosterone, then he or she probably took illegal testosterone.

Because of all the problems with drugs in sports, the number of laboratories that can do these urine tests has increased dramatically. But standard laboratory procedures and accreditation (or examination) programs are also needed. Currently, the International Olympic Committee operates the only formal examination program in the world. The College of American Pathologists is trying to develop a program of its own. Even if a lab has very experienced workers, we do not have all of the standard drugs needed to make a positive identification of some steroids and their metabolites. Since there is so much missing, it is hard to use current procedures to accurately identify many compounds other than testosterone.

The laboratory procedures are getting better every year. Improvement is needed so that urine samples are not incorrectly analyzed. A false positive test is one in which steroids are found in the urine but were not taken by the athlete. Many times an athlete will claim that he or she was given a drink containing a steroid just so they would be disqualified. A false positive test occurs when a steroid looks a lot like another drug that is not banned. For example, some female athletes take birth control pills. When these women test positive for steroids, they claim that the test was a false positive because the machine really found the steroid drug that is in the pill. Angel Myers, an American swimmer, was removed from the U.S. team just before the 1988 Olympic games in Seoul, Korea, because she tested positive for steroids. She claimed that her birth control pill was mistaken for

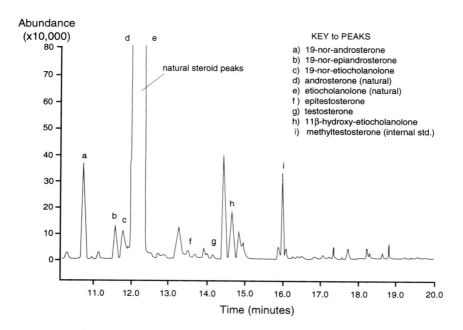

Abundance
(x10,000)

KEY to PEAKS

a) 19-nor-androsterone
b) 19-nor-epiandrosterone
c) 19-nor-etiocholanolone
d) androsterone (natural)
e) etiocholanolone (natural)
f) epitestosterone
g) testosterone
h) 11β-hydroxy-etiocholanolone
i) methyltestosterone (internal std.)

natural steroid peaks

Time (minutes)

A gas chromatograph (GC) reading is shown, tracing of an athlete's urine (for example, a urine screen). Both natural and illegal steroids are shown as peaks which are labeled using the the letters *a* through *i*.

the steroid nandrolone, a banned substance. Laboratories now measure the metabolites of birth control pills in order to prevent false positive tests.

Greater improvements in the laboratory also helped catch Ben Johnson at the 1988 Summer Olympics. The drug that Ben took, stanozolol, could not really be detected four years earlier during the 1984 Games in Los Angeles. Now, both stanozolol and its unique breakdown products can be accurately measured.

Athletes Try to Beat the Tests

However, even if the problems in the laboratory are fixed, there is no guarantee that urine testing will prevent steroid abuse. Many athletes use steroids only during their training periods. The steroids do not have to be in the body during the actual competition. This is because the beneficial effects can be seen for many weeks after the individual has stopped taking the steroid. Some long-lasting injectable steroids could be detected up to six months after a single injection. These are no longer used. Almost all of the urine tests are announced. This means that the athletes know when to stop taking the drugs in order to give themselves time to let the steroids get out of their bodies. Most athletes now stop taking oral steroids two to four weeks and injectable steroids three to six weeks before competing. Athletes are at the greatest risk for being tested during competition. Thus, the athlete can get the beneficial effects of the steroid while reducing the chances of being caught.

Recently, it has been found that some athletes actually send their urine to laboratories for testing while they are training with steroids. They send more samples at various times after they stop taking steroids so they can find out when the steroid is

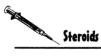

completely removed from their bodies. This helps the athlete predict when he or she should stop taking a particular steroid to avoid being caught.

Scientists need a new method for detecting steroids since it is so hard and expensive to run urine tests on every athlete. One possible solution may be to measure the specific changes that steroids produce in blood tests. However, many different diseases also can change blood values. If this has occurred, then the person might be falsely accused of using steroids. Since steroids change many chemicals in the blood, a positive test for steroids might be seen only when a specific number and type of changes has occurred. This procedure uses tests that are very easy to do. Also, the test results are quickly available. Scientists have looked at a number of possible indicators. These include levels of various chemicals produced by the liver, levels of muscle enzymes, levels of different types of cholesterol, the percentage of red blood cells to plasma (called the hematocrit), the amount of hemoglobin (which helps the blood carry oxygen), levels of various hormones produced by the brain, and, in males, the number of sperm cells. Only the suspicious blood chemistry studies would be followed with the more expensive urine screen for a positive identification. Overall, this plan could be cheaper and would be available to more programs.

Finally, athletes are now using other substances, such as human growth hormone, erythropoietin, and somatomedin. These substances will be even harder to measure in a person. This is because these chemicals are removed from the body very fast (within hours). So these substances may be impossible to detect using the methods that we now have.

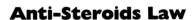

Anti-Steroids Law

In 1990, the U.S. Congress activated a law that now controls the
sale of steroids in the United States. This means that drug companies have to keep very detailed records of which steroids they
make and how much they sell. This level of control is the same as
that used for certain drugs of abuse including Tylenol™ with co-
deine and some amphetamine-like and depressant-like drugs.
Some scientists and lawmakers are upset by this since it now is
more difficult to do research on these drugs. Research is a very
important part of understanding how drugs work. Both animals
and humans are valuable research subjects. As noted in the first
chapter, most of our knowledge about steroids comes from
research with animals.

Sources for Getting Steroids

Most adult and adolescent users get their steroids from the black
market. The black market is an illegal source that often comes
from other countries. Many times, its as easy as sending money
and an order form to a foreign address and receiving steroids in
the mail.

Drug pushers are people who buy and sell drugs. Many
times, they appear at gyms or health clubs. This is because many
of the potential users are working out. Both adults and
adolescents can be drug pushers. These people are breaking the
law. If they are caught, they can be fined and even go to jail.

It is very hard to catch these people who sell steroids. To
catch drugs in the mail, the government has specially trained
dogs. While these dogs can sniff out marijuana, cocaine, and

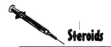

heroin, they cannot smell steroids. Thus, the job of keeping steroids out of adolescents' hands is even harder.

About 20 percent of steroid users get the drugs from a health professional. This means that some doctors, pharmacists, and veterinarians are giving out steroid hormones. More importantly, it means that these professionals may not understand the risks of giving steroids to adolescents. Since there is strong control over the sale of steroids in this country, many athletes use steroids that were made for use in animals. These drugs are not approved for use in humans, and these people are taking a very big risk.

Questions For Discussion

1. Do you think testosterone has value as a legal medication? Give examples to support your answer.

2. What do you think would happen to steroid use among athletes if all urine screens at sporting events were unannounced and could happen any time during the year, including during training periods?

3. Why is it hard to detect illegal testosterone in the body?

4. Why do many of the illegal steroids come from foreign countries?

4

How Do Steroids Work?

The amount of testosterone that the body makes is very small. Males have twenty to sixty times more testosterone than females. Large amounts of testosterone are needed three times during a male's lifetime.[1] The first is when the male is still an embryo in his mother's womb. Testosterone levels increase as he develops male characteristics. The second time is right after the boy is born. The third time is during puberty. This last period of need continues into adulthood. Puberty is that time when the male or female body changes and becomes sexually developed. A boy's voice begins to deepen, and his body hair begins to grow. Also, the boy begins to grow more muscles and to gain weight. The major difference in muscle growth between adolescent males and females is in the shoulders. If the right amount of testosterone is not present during these phases, then the male will not develop properly.

The major female steroid hormone, estrogen, does not increase muscle growth like testosterone. Estrogens are also used to treat certain diseases, but they are not abused. Likewise, other hormones such as thyroid hormone, insulin, and others are not abused. Growth hormone, however, is now being used by some athletes to avoid the problems with steroids.

Steroids Act on the Cells

Scientists have discovered how steroids work. The basic process is the same for the naturally-occurring testosterone as it is for the artificial steroids. Some of these steroids are taken as a pill, and some are injected. First, testosterone is released from the testes and travels through the bloodstream. Since the blood travels everywhere in the body, testosterone can reach every organ. Once it reaches a tissue, the blood takes it very close to the cells. The steroid attaches to the cell by special holding areas called receptors. Once it is attached, the cell draws the testosterone into the cell body. This process is shown in Figure 5.

The testosterone is then transported to the command center of the cell—the nucleus. Here, the cell's machinery begins to run faster and causes new deoxyribonucleic acid (DNA) to be produced. (DNA is the instruction sheet for all of the body's functions.) In fact, DNA is the blueprint for making every person, animal, and plant. The scientists in the movie *Jurassic Park* used the DNA from the blood found inside very old mosquitos to make new dinosaurs. The messages from DNA are converted to new proteins. These new proteins are then

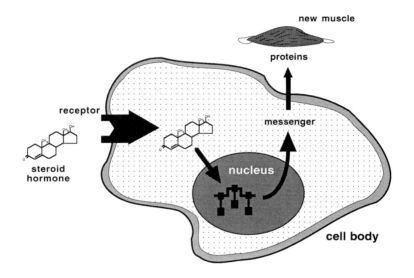

new muscle

proteins

receptor

messenger

nucleus

steroid
hormone

cell body

Figure 5

A testosterone molecule is actively carried into the muscle cell where it
attaches to the nucleus. Once in the "command center" of the cell, it
creates messenger chemicals that trigger the production of new
proteins in the form of muscle or other tissue.

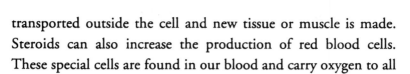

transported outside the cell and new tissue or muscle is made. Steroids can also increase the production of red blood cells. These special cells are found in our blood and carry oxygen to all other tissues.

Tissue-Building Properties of Steroids

The beneficial effects of steroids can occur at many levels. Once in the muscle cells, the steroid causes the normal building processes to speed up. These same effects occur after exercise, only the steroid causes it to happen faster. Muscle normally breaks down when it is strained, as during strenuous exercise. However, the steroid blocks the breakdown of existing muscles. This is called the anti-catabolic effect of steroids. Finally, the steroid helps the body use amino acids for making new muscle protein.

It takes a few days to make new proteins. This is why steroid users take the drugs for many weeks at a time. Any beneficial effects of the steroid are delayed. However, if the person stops taking the steroid, the desired effects will remain for a short while. This is why many athletes train with steroids and then stop taking them a few weeks before competition.

It is important to know that the body is always making and breaking down tissue. This is true for muscle as well. Steroids can increase the production of new protein, but they also block the breakdown of older muscle. These two actions work together to increase muscle size and to increase body weight. This effect to increase size and weight is the major reason that nonathletes (especially adolescents) take steroids.

The natural process of steroid action is very important. Small amounts of testosterone are necessary for proper growth. Steroid abusers think that if small amounts of steroid hormones cause a

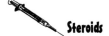

little bit of growth, then large doses should cause greater growth. Now you can understand why people might want to take these drugs. Steroids have similar "desired" effects in males and females.

The undesired effects, however, are different in males and females. These undesired or bad effects are described in later chapters. The most desired effects are an increase in muscle size, increased performance, and an increase in strength.

Both males and females can get these effects from steroids. Another very important effect is that steroids speed up recovery from injury. Ben Johnson, the Canadian sprinter who had his gold medal taken away, hurt his hamstring muscle in May of 1988. This large muscle is the one on the back of the thigh. He received steroids for this injury even though his doctor knew that the Olympic Games would begin in October. However, Johnson probably did not take the steroid just once, because the drug was still in his body by the time he ran his race in October.

Other Effects of Steroids

Since recovery time from injury is shorter after steroids, an athlete can train much harder and longer than someone who is not using these drugs. More training can lead to greater strength. Many football players use steroids to "bulk up" and compete against their opponents. Some athletes claim that they have to take steroids just to keep up with the guys on the other teams.

Another effect of steroids is to increase the number of red blood cells in the blood. These specialized cells carry oxygen to the muscles and to other tissues. Some long-distance runners have used steroids to help them improve their endurance. Greater endurance lets them run longer and farther.

Do Steroids Actually Work?

Scientists disagree over whether steroids actually increase muscle size and improve strength and performance, but this appears to be due largely to the inaccurate manner in which tests were performed in the past. From 1965 to 1977, a total of twenty-five studies were carried out to see if steroids actually increased strength.[2] About one-half of the studies showed some improvement and the other half did not. One of the studies was run by Dr. David Freed and his associates. They conducted a careful study of the effects of steroids on performance in 1975.[3] They found that the weight lifters could lift more weight after taking a steroid. The weight lifters gained weight too. Many of the other studies also found an increase in body weight. This effect is due to an increase in body water and may cause the muscles of some bodybuilders to have a puffy look. It is also possible that the steroids increase aggressive behavior. If a bodybuilder or weight lifter is more aggressive, then he or she may actually train harder. Harder training is one sure way to improve performance.

Many scientists now agree that steroids can increase muscle size and strength, but only if the person eats a high-protein diet and has an intensive exercise program. This makes good sense because we need protein to grow. It appears that steroids work best only in people who have already gained a lot of muscle and strength. The steroids appear to give them just a little bit more. If a person who had never trained with weights before began to exercise and take steroids at the same time, there would be no special effect from the steroids. In fact, that person would gain muscle at the same rate as someone who was not taking steroids.[4]

There are also examples of experiments that have not found

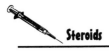

any improvement with steroid use. The failure of many studies to find the effects of steroids was due largely to many flaws in the studies. For example, doses of steroids one-tenth or one-fiftieth as great as those used by actual athletes were used in tests. In addition, the diets and training programs used in the studies did not match those of someone actually lifting weights regularly, and too brief a period of time was often studied. One of the biggest problems with these studies is that the amount of steroids (the dose) given is smaller than what an athlete would use in real life. It would be unethical to give such high doses in a research study. Also, many of the studies did not put the research subjects on a high-protein diet.

Measuring Performance

Performance is very hard to measure. There are many ways that an athlete's performance can be changed. Dr. John Lombardo has outlined the many factors that can affect performance.[5] These include: the level of conditioning, skill, diet, psyche, opponent, environment, sleep, drugs, and genetics.

Conditioning improves with training. The more you train, the better you get. Many people do aerobic exercise to improve their conditioning and stamina. A well-conditioned heart will help the rest of the body perform well. Good muscle endurance means that you can work longer without feeling tired.

Skill is something you learn. It is the ability to do an activity very well. No one is born with the ability to hit a baseball or kick a football. You learn how to do it from someone else. (Of course, some skills are inherited from your parents.) Then, if you practice hitting, catching, or kicking a ball, your skill will increase.

Diet, or nutrition, is another very important factor in performance. Your muscles, like the engine of a car, need fuel to run. A car gets its energy from gasoline. Our bodies get energy from certain foods we eat. Carbohydrates are an excellent source of energy. Protein is needed for building muscle, and even small amounts of fat are needed.

Psyche is the psychological readiness for playing the game. The phrase "getting psyched up" means getting the mind prepared. Performance is best when we concentrate on what we are doing. It would be very hard to hit a baseball if you were thinking about the new compact disk that was just released by your favorite rock star instead of whether the pitcher is throwing a curve ball or a fast ball.

The abilities of your opponent can also affect your performance. Some people play very well against a certain type of player. When I played tennis at Penn State University in the early 1970s, I always played better against opponents who hit the ball hard. If my opponent hit the ball very easy, I found that I took too much time thinking about where to hit the ball, and I often hit it out of the court! I learned this weakness in high school. My very first victory was against someone who could barely hit the ball over the net. It took me almost four hours to beat him. The coach almost called the game because of darkness.

The environment or "home field" can have a big effect on performance. It is always easier to perform in front of supportive spectators. Also, an athlete is more familiar with the home field. Some professional football teams had artificial turf put in their home field. Teams who are used to playing on real grass often have trouble with the field when they come to town.

A good night's sleep is important because both the brain and body need to rest. Without sleep, you begin to feel tired and have trouble concentrating. Sleep or rest also gives the muscles a chance to recover from the effects of training. Another reason that I took so long to beat my opponent was because I could not get to sleep the night before. I was so excited about my very first match that I tossed and turned most of the night. Luckily, the coach made us run two miles every day, so I was in pretty good shape. But boy, was I tired at the end!

Certain types of drugs can either help or hurt performance. Illegal drugs like cocaine and marijuana hurt performance. Alcohol is a depressant drug, so it slows you down, making it hard to compete. Steroids can either help or hurt performance. It depends on how the drugs are used and the sport that is being played.

Your genes can control what is called "natural ability." Since you cannot choose your parents, this is one factor that is out of your control. When I was in high school, I was 5'5" tall and weighed only 105 pounds. My dad was 5'6", and my mom was 5'2". I figured that I would never be a football star. Even though I was a very fast runner, the other guys would have crushed my little body. My mom bought me a tennis racket for my sixteenth birthday. When selecting a sport, it is important to work with your natural strengths. A lightweight body frame is no match for "Bigfoot." I stayed with tennis.

Steroids affect the body in many ways. The various desirable effects that people want from these drugs were described in this chapter. In the next two chapters, the bad and undesirable effects of steroid use will be discussed.

Questions For Discussion

1. Why isn't the female hormone, estrogen, abused like testosterone?

2. What effects do long-distance runners think they get from using steroids?

3. What are some ways of measuring whether steroid hormones actually work?

4. What do you think is the most important factor in athletic performance? Why?

5

Are Steroids Bad for My Body?

There is no question that steroids can hurt your body in many ways. Some of these bad or undesired effects are bothersome and may annoy you, but there is no permanent damage. These are usually called side effects. More severe toxic effects can occur, some of which are permanent. These effects can cause major problems and may even cause death. But not everyone has the same experience with steroids. One athlete can stack six different steroids and have only a bad case of acne. Another person might get very sick on just one steroid. It is important to remember that the number and severity of side effects and adverse effects is based on the dose of the steroid. Higher doses cause more problems. Most of the side effects occur because these drugs have androgenic or male-like effects. Since all muscle-building steroids produce male-like effects, these side effects will always happen. Toxic reactions are due to a direct effect of the steroid on an organ.

Side Effects

Let's talk about the side effects first. Many steroid users think that these are minor and that the extra hassle is worth the results. The side effects are different for males and females. [1,2,3]

Male users can get severe acne and pimples and develop early balding. In addition, their skin and eyes can turn yellow, their breasts can enlarge, and their testicles can shrink. Also, the number of sperm cells made is drastically reduced. The amount of facial and body hair increases, and the hair follicles can become infected. These effects usually go away when the steroid use stops. Interest in sex (called libido) increases at first. As steroid use continues, interest in sex actually decreases.

The side effects in young boys are basically the same except for two important differences. First, if the boy is still growing and takes high doses of steroids, then he will stop growing in height. This is because testosterone-like steroids cause the long bones (the ones that determine height) to stop growing. The second difference is that steroids can cause painful increases in the sexual organs of young boys.

Adolescent boys (and girls) are smaller than adults. For this reason, they may have more side and toxic effects because the drug dose, compared to body size, is very large.

Female steroid users also experience side effects. A woman's voice can get deeper, her breasts shrink in size, and she can start to grow facial hair. Body hair increases, and the skin can become coarse. Her body shape may change to look more like a man's

Oral

Injection

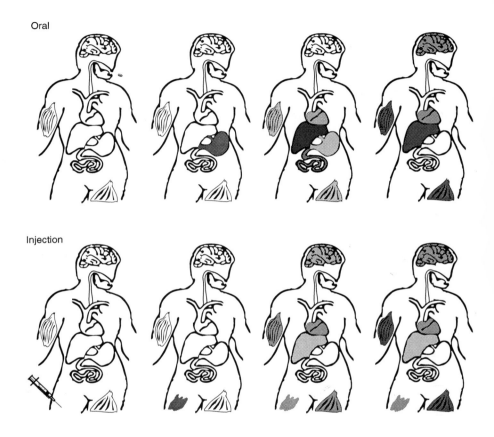

A comparison of how oral and injectable steroids get into the body is illustrated here. The top panel shows how an oral steroid is first absorbed in the stomach and travels to the liver and then finally to the rest of the tissues. The bottom panel shows that an injection of a steroid forms a reservoir depot at the injection site. Then it slowly releases the steroid into the rest of the tissues of the body.

body. Women also lose hair from their heads. The hormonal cycles can also stop, which make it hard for these women to have babies. Unlike the males, some of these changes in females can become permanent after only a few months of taking steroids. Steroids can also have very serious toxic effects on many different body organs. The amount of damage that occurs depends on how much of the steroid is taken. It also appears to be related to which steroids are taken. Usually, the pill forms are more dangerous than the injectable steroids. One reason is that the oral steroids do not last very long so they must be taken every day. Users can inject the liquid steroids once every three or four days. The liquid is usually an oil that can stay in the muscle for a longer period of time. These injectable steroids do not affect the liver as much as the oral preparations. The illustration on page 46 shows how the oral and the injectable steroids get into the body.

Toxic Effects

The toxic or bad effects of steroids change the blood, liver, kidneys, heart, and immune function (infection-fighting ability) and may even increase the chances of getting certain types of cancer. These effects may only happen to a very small percent of steroid users. However, if a toxic effect happens to you, then it is 100 percent! Like the side effects, these effects usually go away after the steroids are stopped. However, some effects on the liver may last a long time.[4,5,6]

Toxic Effects to Your Blood and Heart

Our bodies make both high-density and low-density lipoproteins. These substances are in our blood and move fats from different parts of our body. The low-density lipoprotein cholesterol

47

are the "bad" ones and deposit fats in our arteries. The high-density lipoprotein cholesterol are the "good" ones and remove the "bad" cholesterol from the arteries. Our diet also can change the amount of these substances. We can get heart disease if we have too much of the low density lipoproteins. The high density lipoproteins actually help protect us against the low density lipoproteins. Steroid use can decrease the amount of the high density or "good" lipoproteins. If the amounts of the "protector" are decreased, then the chances of having a heart attack are greater. This effect happens mostly with the steroids that you swallow as a pill and can occur after only a few weeks of use.

There is another bad effect of steroids on the blood. They can cause platelets to clump together. Platelets are special cells found in the blood that stick together whenever we bleed. They keep us from bleeding too long by making our blood clot. This is a very important process if we get a cut or a bruise. But, blood clots inside our blood vessels are very dangerous and can cause a stroke or heart attack.

Steroids can also hurt your heart directly.[7] The fate of Benji Ramirez is one such story.[8] Benji was only seventeen years old and played high school football. He started taking steroids at age fifteen. Two years later, he was dead of a heart attack. The Ashtabula, Ohio, county coroner, Dr. Robert A. Malinowski, believed that the heart attack was caused by Benji's steroid use. The sad truth was that Benji did not take steroids to play better football. One of his closest friends was quoted as saying "Benji was not a diehard football player. He used steroids because he wanted to be big and get girls."[9] Many friends said that they saw Benji inject himself with steroids. Even his nickname was "*Roids.*" One friend said that Benji told her that steroids were making him big. He thought that he would get big some day, "...but he said he needed it now. He said he was speeding up time. He was impatient. He didn't want to wait." Sadly, he will never get the chance to see how big he would grow without steroids.

Oral Steroids and Your Liver

Steroids, mostly the oral ones, also hurt the liver. The liver has over five hundred functions in the body. It helps process our food and stores many important vitamins and minerals such as iron, vitamin A, vitamin B_{12}, and vitamin D. The liver also cleans the blood of any toxins and wastes that are produced by our cells. It is also the main organ that metabolizes or breaks down drugs that we take. Oral steroids are very hard on the liver. Since the steroid doses are so high, the liver cannot keep up and is overworked. As the liver becomes damaged, its liquid, bile, is released into the bloodstream. Bile is normally squirted into your stomach to help you digest fatty foods. But when bile gets in the blood, it makes your skin and the white part of your eyes turn yellow. This problem is called jaundice. There have also been some suspected cases of steroids causing cancer of the liver. Many of these cases were not proven, but the possibility still exists that they are related.[10] A measure of how well the liver is working can be obtained from a blood test. It is called a liver function test. Steroid use causes many of these tests to be abnormal. Again, when steroid use stops, the liver tests usually return to normal. This is the only cure.

Toxic Effects to the Kidneys

The kidneys also clean our blood and remove wastes. They produce a clear fluid called urine. It is stored in our bladders until removed. On rare occasions, steroids can damage the kidneys. This damage makes them work harder. Over time, the kidneys can stop working altogether. The only treatment for kidney disease is to have your blood cleaned by a dialysis machine a couple of times each week. If both kidneys stop working, a kidney transplant from a donor is needed.

Toxic Effects to Your Immune System — Cancer

Our immune system is what helps us fight off infections. Long-term steroid use may decrease our defenses against the thousands of viruses, bacteria, and fungi to which we are exposed. This same immune system also takes care of the occasional cancer cell. The reduction of immune function by steroids may let cancer cells develop.[11]

Although heart disease is the number one killer of adults, cancer is probably feared the most. There have been a number of cases of cancer reported by the press. Most of these were liver cancer, but one was brain cancer. Lyle Alzado was a professional football player. He claimed that the steroids that he took since 1967 caused his brain cancer. He died in May of 1992 of his cancer. Doctors cannot say for sure if steroids caused his cancer. Cancer usually takes a very long time to develop. This is why it is hard to prove that any drug or chemical causes cancer. Steroid users appear to be willing to take that chance.

Steroids and Injuries

Many steroid users appear to believe that steroids help prevent injuries. In fact, steroid use can actually lead to injuries more easily. Muscles grow with the steroid use and exercise. Ligaments

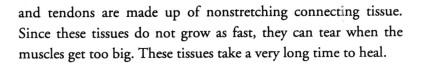
and tendons are made up of nonstretching connecting tissue. Since these tissues do not grow as fast, they can tear when the muscles get too big. These tissues take a very long time to heal.

Counterfeit or Fake Steroids

Steroid abuse has a problem in common with other drugs of abuse. It is difficult to be sure that you are getting true steroids. There are now many counterfeit steroids being sold on the black market.[12] These drugs are made in illegal laboratories and are sold under false advertisement. Some of these drugs are useless and do absolutely nothing. They are a true waste of money. Other counterfeit steroids do contain some active chemicals but may also have impurities. Impurities are substances that do not belong there. Examples of impurities include other chemicals, salt, and other drugs. The danger here is that, just like other drug abuse, the users do not know exactly what they are taking. In fact, many of the above side effects and toxic reactions could be caused from these impurities.

Dangerous Reactions to Steroids

There have been reports of steroid users dying unexpectedly. In 1987, Birgit Dressel of West Germany died of a massive allergic reaction to the drugs she was taking. Many of these were steroids. She had a very severe allergic reaction called anaphylactic shock. A person can be allergic to most anything, but bee stings are the most common. You may know of someone who is allergic to penicillin or some other substance. Many people die each year from bee stings because they are allergic to the venom. King Menes of Egypt died over four thousand five hundred years ago from a wasp sting. This type of allergic reaction does not occur

51

after the first time a person is stung or injected. Instead, the first time the drug is taken, the body is made more sensitive. The bad reaction can occur after the next dose or after a number of doses. Sometimes, only a mild reaction occurs. This usually causes a fever, hives (bumps on the skin), aches and pains, and a cold sweat. In the severe reaction, the person stops breathing. This type of reaction to steroids is rare, but because there are many types of unknown black market products, you do not know what you are getting for your money.

Injecting drugs has its own dangers. The syringe, needle, and solution must all be very clean. Counterfeit injectibles may have lots of bacteria in them, since they are probably not made under sterile conditions. If they are dirty or have bacteria in them, then a local infection can occur. The bacteria can live deep inside the muscle and grow. If left untreated, it becomes infected and can cause a lot of pain and discomfort. There is another danger of injecting drugs. Many times, users share syringes and needles. The AIDS virus can be spread this way. In fact, the first case of a bodybuilder who got AIDS from a shared needle was reported in 1984.[13] Other cases will likely follow, making steroid abuse just as dangerous as heroin abuse.

Questions For Discussion

1. Why do you think oral steroids are more toxic to the body than the ones that are injected?

2. Why do you think side effects and toxic reactions are generally greater in adolescents than in adults?

3. Why do you think some of the negative effects of steroids last longer than others?

4. Which do you think is a greater danger from using steroids: liver damage or cancer? Give reasons for your answer.

5. Why are steroid users at a greater risk of contracting AIDS?

6

Will Steroids Make Me Crazy?

There are many stories in the newspapers and on the news that describe steroid users who will just "snap and go crazy." In general, this usually means that the person becomes very violent and angry at everyone and everything around him or her. However, there are now some reports that steroids do cause some effects that look like certain types of mental disease. Steroid users also may get depressed after their steroid use has stopped. This effect will be discussed in the next chapter on the addictive properties of steroids.

Steroids and Mental Illness

Mania is a type of psychiatric disease. People who have mania are very hyperactive. They move around a lot and talk very fast. They often do many different things—all at the same time! There have been many cases of mania in bodybuilders who use

Off Steroids

Depressed

Panic

None

On Steroids

Psychotic

Manic

Depressed

None

These pie graphs show the proportion of body builders who develop psychiatric symptoms while off steroids (left side) compared to those who develop symptoms while on steroids (right side). Data are extracted from interviews with forty-two body builders.

steroids.[1,2] Steroids may also cause effects that look like schizo-phrenia.[3,4] People with this disease often hear voices and think other people are "out to get them." This type of behavior is also called paranoia.

Mania has been reported in a controlled scientific study. The authors of the study gave either placebo, low-dose, or high-dose methyltestosterone.[5] The steroids were given for only a few days, but some subjects developed mania.

Steroids and Aggressive Behavior

It is clear that steroids can affect your brain. They also can change your behavior. Some steroid users, especially football players want to be more aggressive. They probably think that this helps them play better football. Other athletes think that steroids boost confidence and motivation. These behavioral effects may help them train longer and harder. But the aggressive behavior cannot be turned on and off like a lamp. Behavioral changes can erupt at any time. Problems occur when people are too aggressive at the wrong time. The aggressive and violent behavior can develop in many different ways. Sometimes the person hits people or breaks things. Other times, a male steroid user may bother a female in a sexual way. These behavioral changes can be very scary to the steroid user as well as those around him or her.

Scientists have asked weight lifters how they feel both on and off steroids. In one survey, over half of the men reported that steroids made them more irritable.[6] They were also more aggressive on the drugs. They got into a lot more arguments and even had many more fights during this time. In another survey of female athletes, eight out of ten of the women felt that steroids made them more aggressive.[7] Six of the women liked this because it made them train harder. Another survey found that over 30 percent of the steroid users noticed behavioral changes while they were on steroids.[8] These reports are based on what the steroid user tells the doctors. It is possible that some do not tell the truth. However, it is likely that steroids can cause changes in behavior. The amount of change is based on the amount of steroids that is taken.

Increased aggressive behavior has been called "roid rage" by the media. This term describes an uncontrollable fit of anger or aggressive behavior. For example, Drs. Harrison G. Pope and David L. Katz have treated a number of steroid users who have become very hostile and experienced rage after taking high doses of steroids. They described three cases in a recent paper.[9] One case involved a thirty-two-year-old man. He began to lift weights at age twenty-seven. He was happily married and worked full time as a prison guard. At age thirty, he started to take steroids. He did five cycles of steroids. He also stacked two or three different steroids. Each cycle lasted six weeks. He noticed that he was more irritable and aggressive when he took the drugs. During the fifth cycle, he began to show signs of a type of psychiatric illness called mania. He was hyperactive and felt that nothing could hurt him. But he also grew suspicious of the inmates at the prison and of his wife.

He had car trouble one day and stopped to use a phone at a store. The woman in the store joked that she should charge the guards to use her phone. For the rest of the day, the man became more and more angry at what the woman said. He was so upset that he could not sleep that night. The next morning he drove back to the store and forced the woman into his car. He later said that he only wanted to scare her because of what she had said to

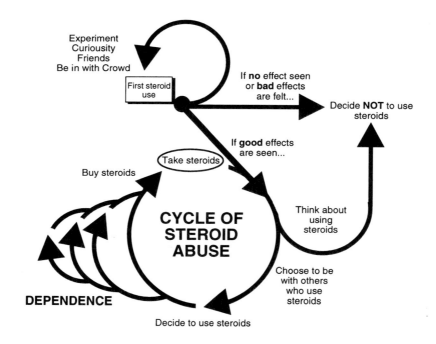

This diagram shows the cycle of steroid use and abuse. The reason why an individual begins taking steroids is not the same reason why he or she continues to take them. There are many decisions that must be made during this process, before abuse begins.

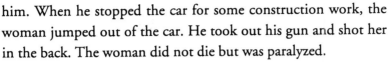
him. When he stopped the car for some construction work, the woman jumped out of the car. He took out his gun and shot her in the back. The woman did not die but was paralyzed.

The man was arrested and put in jail. His steroid supply was gone, and he went through withdrawal. He became very depressed and even thought of committing suicide. The judge sentenced him to twenty years in prison for shooting the woman.

The second case described by Drs. Pope and Katz involved a twenty-three-year-old man. He had started lifting weights at age eighteen and wanted to be in a bodybuilding contest at age twenty-one. He was very quiet and shy before taking steroids. During his first cycle, he used three different steroids at the same time for five months before the competition. He stopped for a few weeks and then started again. This time, he used higher doses. While on the steroids, he noted that his temper became very bad, and he would get into arguments with his parents. He reported that "he would bite chunks out of aluminum cans and tear telephones off the wall." He said that he did this to frighten the people around him. One night, while with two friends, he ripped a telephone booth from its base. He and his friends were in the parking lot of a store. Later on that night, he suggested that they pick up a hitchhiker just to give him a hard time. They drove to some woods where he began to hit the hitchhiker in the back with a 2"x 4" wooden board and then kicked him. The hitchhiker died later that night.

This man was arrested and received a life sentence plus thirty years. During the trial he was shy, and while in prison, he is shy, quiet, and cooperates totally with the prison staff. He says that he is still stunned by the memory of that night.

The third case also involved a young man. He started lifting weights in high school while he trained to play football. He was a local hero, being the first in his high school class to go to college. He even received a scholarship. At age twenty, he started taking steroids. His cycles lasted from six weeks to sixteen months. He usually stopped for about twelve weeks between cycles. His behavior changed from mild-mannered to very irritable while on steroids. He was teaching school at the time, so the change in his behavior was very serious. He even began to take a shotgun out in the car with him and shoot at moving trucks or lights.

His girlfriend broke off their engagement while he was in the last month of a thirteen month-cycle. At first, he did not care that she left him. Later, he planned to kill her with a bomb. With the help of a friend, he placed the bomb under her car. The bomb exploded while she was in the car, but luckily she was not hurt. At the trial, he was sentenced to twenty-two years in prison.

Dr. Pope was involved with another well-known case. This story is about a shy boy who started taking steroids at the age of fourteen. He was being bullied by the other, bigger boys, so he started taking testosterone. Very soon after starting his first cycle, he was arrested for starting a fight. In the next year and a half, he was arrested another three times for fighting. One day, he completely destroyed his room in a fit of rage. His mother took him to the emergency room because she was afraid. She did not know her son was taking steroids. This behavior continued for two years until he was sixteen years old.

One day, he became very angry with his girlfriend. He was jealous and thought she was dating other boys behind his back. He had also drunk some alcohol that day. He then went to his mother's kitchen and got a knife. He asked his girlfriend to go out into the woods with him where he supposedly stabbed her in the back and cut her throat. Her body was found sometime later, hidden in a pond. He was caught, went to court, and was found guilty of murder. He is now in prison for life with no chance for getting out.

Steroids and Suicide

Tommy Chaikin is a steroid user who played football for South Carolina. His use of steroids caused many people a great deal of pain and almost cost Tommy his life. A few years ago, he told his story of violent behavior and near suicide to *Sports Illustrated* magazine.[10] He used steroids for about three years and became very aggressive while on steroids. He was one of the meanest players on the team. His aggression was aimed at everyone, including his teammates and coaches. Once, he got mad at another linebacker just because the linebacker cut in front of him. He quickly threw his teammate to the ground. Then Tommy pulled the guy's helmet up and punched him in the eye. On another day, Tommy had an argument with one of his trainers and was sent to the locker room. When Tommy went back to his locker, he ripped the door off its hinges. Then he went home and used a baseball bat on his refrigerator. After it was broken, he ripped the telephone off the wall. One night, Tommy got drunk. The combination of steroids and alcohol was just too much. That night, he pointed a loaded shotgun at the man who delivered the pizza. Tommy thought it was funny.

Unfortunately, Tommy developed some health problems. He developed tumors on his chest and hands. The doctors thought they were related to the steroids. He also had high blood pressure and got a few injuries to his feet and toes. He was so sick

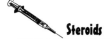

that he quit the team. But he then asked the coach to let him back on the team. Just before his senior year at college, Tommy began to have more serious psychological effects. He felt anxious and nervous. Tommy described the experience this way:

> *... I was starting to battle anxiety attacks that I was sure were caused by steroids. I can't really describe an attack, except to say that it's like your mind is a car engine stuck in neutral with the gas pedal to the floor, just screaming.*[11]

The problems got worse and worse. Tommy started to think about killing himself. He even held a loaded revolver just under his chin. His father's voice from outside his room was the only thing that kept him from pulling the trigger.

There are other examples of steroids causing violent behavior. A thirty-two-year-old bodybuilder murdered his common-law wife while he was taking two different steroids.[12] Other scientists have talked about whether steroid use can cause temporary insanity. If it does, can this effect be used as a defense during a trial for murder?[13] This is a very hard question to answer.

Steroids and Sexual Behavior

Aggressive sexual behavior may be related to testosterone. Violent rapists have very high levels of testosterone.[14] The levels found in the rapists in some studies were much higher than those in other men. A study by Dr. Howard Moss and his colleagues found that steroid users had more desires for sexual contact.[15] These men were also more aggressive and violent. These behaviors can be dangerous combinations that could lead to date rape. The date may start out fine, but later on, the male may want to force his intentions on his companion. Date rape has become a problem for many females, both young and old. Tommy Chaikin also claimed that his sex drive was very strong while he was on steroids.

Unpredictable Reactions

These examples show what steroids can do to some people. Many of these people were pretty shy and quiet before taking steroids. Scientists think that these drugs may change their brains. This effect does not seem to be related to genetics because one of Dr. Pope's patients, the prison guard who shot the store clerk, has an identical twin brother. The twin does not use steroids, and he has not had any episodes of aggression. But you should remember that many successful athletes are very motivated to play hard and win. Some would say you have to be a little crazy to train so hard. Maybe the steroids also push some people over the edge. Does this mean that everyone who uses steroids will become crazy and kill people? No, of course not. But it is possible that some people are more sensitive to the effects of steroids. A steroid user may be fine one minute but then react very differently and become angry over nothing. This is what makes steroids so dangerous.

Questions For Discussion

1. Why do you think aggressive behavior has become so important in our society?

2. Do you think there are times when aggressive behavior is necessary?

3. Do you think that a steroid abuser who kills someone in a fit of rage should be classified as insane and therefore not be punished for the crime?

7

Are Steroids Addictive?

Recently, steroids have been in the newspapers because of some highly publicized news stories. Some users have claimed that they cannot stop using them. They say that they are addicted to them. For many years, people thought that a drug addict was someone who hung out at inner city street corners just to buy "dope." After their purchase, they would quickly run to the nearest public bathroom and inject the drugs directly into their veins. They might even use the water from the toilet to mix up their drugs. Steroid users do not fit this description. However, this is also not a true description of drug addiction in general. This is also why the word addiction is not very useful now. It can mean different things to different people. So, before the addictive properties of steroids can be discussed, the term "addiction" must be better defined.

Definitions of Abuse

The word "addiction" has been used for many years. It was always used to describe habitual use of well-known drugs of abuse such as heroin, cocaine, alcohol, and nicotine. A drug addict was someone who could not stop using a drug. If he or she did stop, they would get very sick. Drug addiction has now been divided into two parts so that it can be better understood.[1] The first part is called abuse liability, and the second part is called dependence.

Abuse liability refers to the actions a person takes to get drugs. This is also called drug-seeking behavior. Simply asking other people where to buy drugs is a type of abuse liability. It means that the person is interested in using them. Buying the drug is the next step in abuse. Finally, actually using the drug is the highest form of abuse liability.

Steroids clearly have an abuse liability. That is, people actively seek them out for desired effects. Many steroid users have lost the ability to stop using the drugs. These individuals believe that they are not big or strong enough. These beliefs may help continue the steroid-seeking behavior. This belief about their body also occurs in junior and senior high school students. One-fourth of the male high school seniors who reported using steroids would not stop taking them even if it were proven that steroids caused liver cancer, permanent sterility, or early heart attacks.[2]

People try drugs for many different reasons. Usually it is to be "in with the crowd" because of peer pressure to try them or to experiment with them and see what they are like. Some people use a drug once or twice and then stop. These people usually decide that it is not for them. Most of the time they do not get the desired effect, or they have a bad effect. However, some people will continue to use drugs. The reasons they continue to use the drugs are very different than why they tried them in the first place. Drugs like heroin, cocaine, alcohol, and nicotine are

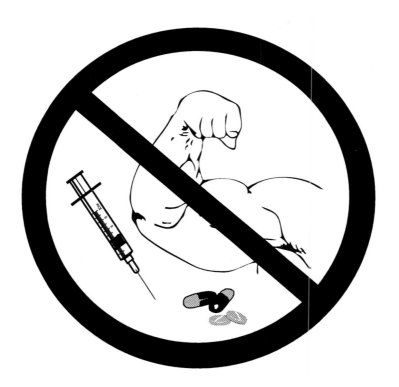

Peer pressure can be a very strong factor in a young adult's decision whether or not to begin using steroids. As this diagram indicates, deciding never to start is the right decision, but it may not be the easiest one.

reinforcing for some people. This means that these drugs make them feel good. Some people call these effects a "rush," "high," or "buzz." These effects only last a very short time. The person must use the drugs again and again to get the same effect. However, the body adapts to these drugs. This is called tolerance.

Steroids are not taken like other drugs of abuse. Most users do not feel the effects of the steroid right after the pill or injection. The steroids can get to the cells of the body rather quickly, but their effects take time to develop.[3] There is also a large placebo effect with steroids. A placebo is an inactive substance. Placebo responses are probably due to expectations or wishful thinking. Placebo responses also occur with the more common drugs of abuse. It is harder to detect an active steroid from an inactive one because the desired effects take so long to develop. In fact, there was a study conducted in 1972 to test whether athletes could detect the effects of steroids.[4] The subjects were told that they would receive steroids. Instead, they were actually given placebo injections. They could not tell that they were given a placebo. It was interesting that their performance improved while receiving the placebo.

Dependence on Steroids

After the person uses the drug a few times, he or she must increase the dose in order to get the same effect. After using a drug for some time, the person becomes dependent on it. Now, their bodies are used to the drug and need the drug in order to function. This means that the person will get sick if he or she stops taking the drug. This is called drug withdrawal. For many drugs, the withdrawal effects include nausea, vomiting, diarrhea, heartburn, muscle cramps, lack of appetite, frequent need to urinate, dizziness, sweating, inability to fall asleep at night, irritability, and painful joints. Withdrawal from alcohol can cause convulsions and even death.

The evidence that steroids cause dependence has only recently been reported. These case reports have found that a number of withdrawal signs appear after the steroid use is stopped.[5,6] In a survey of forty-nine male weight lifters, Dr. K.J. Brower and his colleagues found that the most frequently reported withdrawal signs were steroid craving (52 percent), fatigue (43 percent), depressed mood (41 percent), restlessness (29 percent), no appetite (24 percent), difficulty in falling asleep (20 percent), decreased interest in sex (20 percent), and headaches (20 percent).[7] Similar findings were reported in another study.[8] The results of these studies must be checked to be sure they are representative of other steroid users. However, there has not been a single case of steroid dependence in women or among patients who have been prescribed these drugs for medical reasons. These findings suggest that steroid dependence may not be very common.

Steroid dependence does appear to exist in some people. Treating this problem will be a real challenge for doctors.[9] However, the biggest problem in treating steroid dependence will be in making the diagnosis. Bodybuilders are very secretive about their drug use. Also, these drugs are now banned from competition and are regulated by the Drug Enforcement Agency (DEA). Thus, individuals may not easily admit to using steroids. Doctors must use many tools including physical, mental, and laboratory exams to identify a steroid abuser.[10] Since steroid dependence is so new, there are no guidelines for treating the problem. Doctors are now trying to provide education on the effects of steroids. Suggesting other ways of training without steroids is also very important. Some steroid abusers may need medications to help them through the withdrawal. A combination of the above will be needed to prevent the individual from using steroids again.[11] These treatment plans are the same as those that are used for other drugs of abuse.

Questions For Discussion

1. Why do you think steroids are so frequently abused even though they do not produce a "high" like other drugs?

2. How important do you think the placebo response is to taking steroids?

3. Do you think you would be able to tell if one of your friends was going through withdrawal from steroids? Support your answer with facts.

8

An Interview with a Former Steroid Abuser

Adam Frattasio is a former steroid abuser. He is thirty-one years old, weighs 170 pounds, and still looks very muscular. He was caught selling steroids in 1986, just before the laws changed. He has been off steroids since September 14, 1984, but still works out in the gym. Since 1986, he has been talking to young people about the dangers of steroid use and abuse.[1]

Author: Thank you for agreeing to be interviewed. It looks like this is very good timing since I see that you have an article in one of the muscle magazines.[2] When did you first start using steroids?

Frattasio: I first started using them just as I turned eighteen. I used for four years.

Author: How did you learn about steroids in the first place?

Frattasio: I would say that almost everybody who eventually takes steroids learns about them from the magazines. Bodybuilders are curious, even if the articles are negative. So everybody, we're talking the early 80s which is before the public was really keyed in, knew they were out there, and we wondered about them.

Author: How did you start taking steroids?

Frattasio: I was working in a health club selling memberships and training people. One of the older guys that worked with me told me about his brother who played college football. He went to a local doctor and got a prescription for a drug called Winstrol™, which I didn't know what it was at the time, of course. It made it sound so much easier to get now. It wasn't just in the magazines, it was five miles down the street for a $10 prescription price - a check-up. Back then it was a lot easier. Things have changed a lot now. But, being of an experimentative nature anyways, the type of a person that would try things, I gave it a shot. I had college approaching, I was only 125 pounds at the time. I was very strong, I had a 230-pound bench press at that weight, too. I was in shape, but that is tiny.

Author: So you had been working out?

Frattasio: Oh yeah, I worked out for two years. Like a maniac, I mean nutty. Three times a day sometimes. So I was really into it. So I wasn't just some clown deciding that he wanted to get big over the summer. I wanted to put on some weight, so I got them [the steroids].

Author: Did you want to play football or other sports at all?

Frattasio: No, I played hockey and baseball in college, but they [steroids] weren't for sports because I was good enough—I was a starter in high school. I was good enough without them. I wanted the physical look and the performance. I took lifting weights as a sport on its own, and I wanted to get as good as possible. I ended up competing so I took them for that reason also. But the physical size and performance—that's why I took them—not for the sports I was playing.

Author: In what sports did you compete?

Frattasio: In bodybuilding and power lifting. Every power lifter, everybody who lifts weights, wants to look good, and personally, I don't have the genetics to be a good bodybuilder. I'm small and thin. I entered a couple of contests, didn't do that well, and found that I was a lot stronger than some of my friends who started out as power lifters and didn't have the strength. They looked better.

Author: They looked better but didn't have the strength?

Frattasio: I was the opposite, I was strong as hell and really didn't look it. So I went the other way, [went into power lifting, not bodybuilding] and I did fairly well at a competitive level.

Author: How much improvement in your performance did you see? How much additional weight could you lift?

Frattasio: I pretty much have that down year-to-year, cycle-to-cycle. I remember it all. During the first three months of steroids, I gained fifteen pounds [of] body weight. Now, fifteen pounds may not sound like a lot to a guy who weighs 400 pounds, but for a 125-pound guy, you know that's probably more. My bench press went from a 230 to 275 which wasn't bad. Now I would stop using steroids for baseball. So baseball was kind of a cleaning out time. I played only one year of hockey in college, and that was a clean out too, so that didn't really matter... And then the gains went up from there. As far as body weight goes, the first fifteen pounds was the biggest. And actually that first gain was probably the biggest when my body hit the steroids, it was probably like a dry sponge in a rainstorm. Every year after that I would gain about ten pounds. The following year, I came to college at 150; the year after that, I came to my junior year at 160; and the year after that, 170. The lifts went up progressively. I was on the squat which approached 600 pounds at 159 pounds bodyweight! In fact, I was the strongest of my life at 159 pounds and in my third year on steroids, also taking human-growth hormone. Actually, it wouldn't be called a steroid. But I was taking all kinds of 'roids with it. So, 560 squat at 159 pounds and I tore ligaments and broke my knees. I was going for the 600, and I fell short of that because of injuries. The bench press topped out at 365, and I tore a pec, so that took care of that. And all those injuries are still there to this day.

Author: Could you think back and tell me how you felt just before you took that first Winstrol™ pill?

Frattasio: I got them in August, and I was due to go to college in early September. I went to Framingham State. I held them, I didn't want to take them yet. It was almost like this magic thing of I will wait 'till my whole new life started. My whole new life in college and my whole new life as this big person on steroids. Those two weeks that I waited before I took them was almost like having a spare $100 bill that you can spend anytime you want. You got to keep yourself from taking it. It was great, it was like having a Christmas present two weeks early in the closet. I finally started taking them, but they didn't work right away. I was really depressed.

I had some placebo effects as far as strength goes, but I was really interested in getting bigger because I was so small and the weight just wasn't coming. After the bottle was almost done, close to the end of September, I said "Well, obviously steroids are like everything else they sell in the magazines: They talk them up and they don't really work!" I decided that I would finish out the bottle and forget it and chalk it up as an experiment. I was going to do that, but over one weekend as the pills were finished I gained 5 pounds in two days! Over the previous four years, I gained 5 pounds a year. I mean I was a 100-pound freshman in high school, then 115 and then 120 and then graduating at 125. So five pounds in two days was amazing to me, and I said, "Oh, yeah." It just took a little while to kick in, but they're here. And then all of a sudden, bang another couple of pounds every week, and the bench pressing went up 240, 250, 260, and then finally 275. Of course, I bought a couple of more bottles. I finished off the cycle 'till my freshman year of baseball.

Author: So they worked for you?

Frattasio: Yeah.

Author: Have you ever used the injectable steroids?

Frattasio: Yeah.

Author: Can you tell me a little bit about that first experience with a needle? Isn't it a little different to take a pill than it is to give yourself an injection?

Frattasio: It is initially if you've never done it, but once you've done it, there is no difference. When I first took the pills, I knew that they were bad. You know steroids are bad. You know any kind of a medication that you take for not a medical reason is bad. Or at least I understood that. I wasn't a dummy. Although after you hear my stories, you'll think I'm a dummy.

But, when I took Winstrol™, I said, "Okay I'll take this drug, but I will not take the stronger drug Dianabol™ because that's dangerous." Even though Winstrol™ is probably just as dangerous. There was an older fellow that started working at my hometown gym, so when I came back from college to live back at home, this guy who was an older power lifter introduced me to Dianabol™. He said, "If you really want to get strong, you'll take Dianabol™." That's all I have to hear. All I need is somebody just to nudge me a little bit, and I'll do anything just to get big and strong. So he got me on Dianabol™ and I remember saying to myself, "Yeah, okay, I'll take Dianabol™, but I'll never shoot myself. I'll never inject myself." And sure enough, if you really want to get big, you're gonna—you know—here you go the testosterone injections and bang, go ahead, shoot me in my tricep.

I remember it was at a gas station. It was me and

another friend of mine. He was a year younger than me, and he got me in the tricep. It was no big deal... I mean, if he told me to eat cow [____] and said that it would make me get big, I would have done it—no problem. When I went back to college, he would send me syringes and steroids. He was making some money off of me. After a while, I figured that out, and I just learned how to do it myself. Then I got into the black market and got my own. The injections were no big deal.

Author: You had no hesitation?

Frattasio: Not at all. In fact, the hardest thing to do was to get needles. They shouldn't have been at the time, but they were. Six months later they weren't. But we would use the same needle over and over again. Before AIDS and all that.

Author: This was in the early '80s?

Frattasio: Yeah, I remember using a needle, oh, fifteen times. It would be so dull that I would have to get myself up against a wall, stick the needle in my butt, and ram the plunger up against the wall to get it in. And then, of course, we would light them on fire to try to sterilize them. We got so psychologically addicted to the drugs. I was used to taking my shot Friday morning and in the afternoon I'd bench. If I didn't take that shot Friday morning, I wouldn't have a good bench. It was just a psychological thing.

Author: So you used them once a week?

Frattasio: At least, at first, it was once a week. I didn't go crazy on doses like most of my other friends did. My abuse was staying on too long. There's three ways of abusing the drugs: to use them in the first place without a medical reason, to take too much, and to stay on too long. I stayed on too long.

Author: There is a lot of controversy over whether steroids work. Where would you be now if you had never taken steroids but still continued to workout at the same pace?

Frattasio: I remember about ten years ago when I was still taking steroids. A pretty good drug-free power lifter in the gym was trying to convince me that I could get just as strong if I didn't use the drugs, and I just laughed at him. Now, he was probably 80 percent correct. I'm very strong now, I can squat over five hundred pounds right now, maybe five hundred fifty pounds right now. I cannot bench press more than three hundred pounds. My shoulders are gone; my pecs hurt me.

Author: But you had the injury to your chest muscle.

Frattasio: Yeah. So I think if I never did the steroids and never had the injuries, maybe my bench press could be better today. My knees still bother me; those little tendons that I ripped still bother me. So maybe I could be better or just as good (as if I had never done steroids). We're talking a lot of training time that I put in over the past, say nine years that I've been drug-free. That's not typical of the steroid user. I'm just a very motivated person.

Author: Let's talk a little bit about the side effects of steroids. You said earlier that your insides "started to go."

Frattasio: I would start 'roiding in May through September all through the summer right into the next college year. This happened for three straight years, the same exact thing. In late September, my insides started to hurt. The only way I could describe it, I felt like my organs were sick, were swollen. I could almost picture them filled with pus and yellowed. My eyes, around my eyes, as yellowish, my skin looked weird. It was a feeling of unwellness and I knew that was time to get off, so I would always get off for October. Clean out for October, get right back on until the baseball season started again in February.

Author: What else?

Frattasio: As far as the other physical things, after the first full year on it, I started with the gynecomastia [enlarged breasts], and soreness in my chest. In fact, it's come back now for some reason. I don't know why. If I squeezed my nipples, a sticky substance would come out, which I don't really know what it is or what it was. Of course, the older power lifter, Joe, told me, "Don't worry about it, it will go away." Urination frequency. I went nuts, to the point of passing out. I'd urinate an amazing amount. I remember almost passing out a few times while on the subway and not being able to get off. After my first contest, I overdosed on methyltestosterone. I took forty of them before my first squat. I urinated blood for three days after that and started passing scabs through my urinary tract. Ever since that day, I have a problem urinating. It felt like I was urinating acid. It was something, and then the blood would come out like cranberry juice. It was funny, but that scared me off for a couple of weeks. But right when I started losing the weight, I got right back on.

Author: What about black market steroids? Weren't you worried about taking something that you didn't know what was in it?

Frattasio: Not back then. I mean there were all kinds of steroids out there that were legal and legitimate. It's like using one brand of soap, or another. It's still soap, and it was the same thing. The problem is after 1987 when the Feds cracked down. It became harder to get steroids from the legitimate places like pharmaceutical warehouses. You can't do that anymore. There is a lot of money to be made, so now you are getting bogus drugs. That's the problem. The Feds say that at least 50 percent of what you buy now is bogus. I agree. Because, during the tail end of my selling days, I was selling all fake stuff—and I didn't even know it.

Author: You have been talking to kids about steroids the past few years. There are a lot of thirteen-and fourteen-year-olds out there thinking about trying steroids. What do they know about them, and why do they want to use them at such an early age?

Frattasio: Well, nobody was taking steroids in junior high in the early '80s. Very few in high school, very few. It was unheard of. Now it is. The attitudes of these thirteen-and fourteen-year-old kids now is the same that I had when I was eighteen. They want to get big and strong. They've heard that these things can do it and they don't believe the doctors who say they don't work. They don't believe that

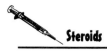

so they also don't believe that these things cause major side effects. Plus they don't care. When I was eighteen, I didn't care whether I lived or died as long as I was big in my coffin. You can't tell a thirteen-year-old kid don't do this because when you're thirty you might die of heart disease. Thirty to a thirteen-year-old kid is light-years away. When you think about it, when do you need size? You need it as a teenager and in college. Now, I'm thirty-one and I'm going to have a kid in a month. I don't care, you know, about how big I am or how strong I am. I care about my kid.

Author: So what do you tell them when they ask you about steroids?

Frattasio: I come from a family of nine athletes. I'm the second oldest, so most of them have grown up with it, and only one has taken steroids. The rest of them have not. And one of them was drug-free as a champ—an All-American power lifter with national records. Now, I say to myself, "Why did they not go my route?" And I think its because they had the truth. They saw it for what it was, and they didn't want to go the way I did. But I really think you have to go with the truth on these kids and then leave it up to them. Everybody is different. Some will get the bad effects, some will not.

Author: Are the social pressures different now?

Frattasio: It's not as acceptable in society right now to take them. Society, as a whole, is like a blanket over steroids and if you take steroids now you're frowned upon. In the early '80s, there was no awareness of their dangers and nobody really gave a damn. It's a whole different attitude now. And I think that's the thing when you change society's attitudes about things. And the pressure of society is big. I wouldn't want to be on steroids right now because of the society. I wouldn't want to be looked upon as a guy on 'roids right now. That pressure wasn't around back then.

Author: Things have really changed that much?

Frattasio: They have. I think as much as I fault the media for putting me on steroids, I guess I can also look at the media as creating the shroud. And it's there. It changes a lot of things. There's a big drug-free movement in the contests now. That's very important too. There are many more drug-free contests to enter now for athletes as an avenue to express their athletic endeavors than there were when I was doing them. And now, you get more of a pat on the back for going the drug-free way.

Author: What about the kids who are not doing them for sports?

Frattasio: With those kids, they fall under that shroud with their parents and even kids in school. The majority of kids in school, let's face it, aren't going to do steroids, and they look down on steroids. And now if you walk through school with some muscles, even if you are drug-free, they say "Oh he's taking steroids, he's on 'roids." And you're not cool, it's just not cool.

Adam wrote an article for Muscular Development. It ended with this:

I worked very hard for my gains—both on and off

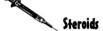

drugs—but the steroid-augmented results were not real or lasting. Such gains are tied to a dependence that can dictate—and ultimately ruin—your life. If you are on—GET OFF! If you are thinking of trying steroids—DON'T! Look in the mirror; for better or worse, that is who you are. Work hard naturally and you will be the ultimate winner in the long run. Take it from one who knows.[3]

Questions For Discussion

1. Do you think that articles in bodybuilding and fitness magazines help or make the problem worse?

2. Why do you think that the risk of physical injury is so high among steroid users?

3. How can you tell if the steroids that you are buying are real or fake?

4. How do you think the media could help the steroid problem?

2

Society and Steroids?

The social effects of steroid use involve your friends, family, and other people around you. You may have heard the phrase, "It's not whether you win or lose, it's how you play the game." This is a basic principle of sports. However, sporting events are now big business. The owners of professional teams can make a lot of money. Just look at the amount of money many professional athletes make. Some of them make millions of dollars for a three- or four-year contract. It is this desire to win and increase personal gain that pushes people to use any method to improve their chances of success. These people want to win at all costs—even above fair play.

Learning Values

But where does this all start? Since we learn many of our values from our family, some think that the desire to win is shaped very

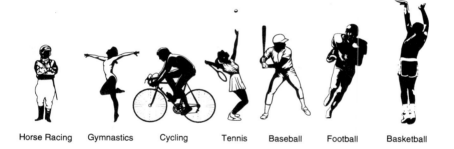

Horse Racing   Gymnastics   Cycling   Tennis   Baseball   Football   Basketball

Certain body frames are best suited for certain sports.

early in life. The interest in getting big can be changed by the people around you. These include your family, friends, and those with whom you work out. In the interview with Adam Frattasio, he commented on this topic.[1]

Frattasio: I have this aunt. Every time she'd see me off steroids (I had lost weight, you know), she would say, "Adam, you look so good, you lost weight." Now, that's the worst thing that you could tell somebody like me. I would go right back [on steroids] again. Or someone in the gym would say, "Gee, you used to bench 350 pounds, what happened?" or "You used to be big, what happened?" Stuff like that works on your psyche, and you refuse to get off.

Author: Do adults influence a young person to use steroids?

Frattasio: When I was working in a gym, there was a father from my hometown whose son was coming up. He was one of those controlling fathers. He'd say, "I want to get my son to play this, and you're going to play that..." He wanted me to put his fifteen-year-old son on steroids so he'd be bigger for the high school football team. I remember another kid from Central Mass who was going to Michigan to play football telling me that "Yeah, the coach said I don't know if I'll play as a freshman, but if I could put on twenty or thirty pounds.... You know, can you help me out?"

I remember a kid who was spending years and years down in the East Coast hockey league, the slapshot league. He was a little center. A professional hockey team came up to him and said, "If you could just come in twenty pounds heavier..." The kid went on steroids; he had to go on steroids. He was in the East Coast league for four years, you know, and he has a chance for the Chicago Black Hawks. Of course, he never made it, but it's powerful.

Author: Did everyone in your family know that you were using steroids? How did your parents and brothers and sisters take it?

Frattasio: In the early '80s [when I used steroids], the general population had no idea what steroids were, and they didn't give a damn. They didn't until the mid-'80s, and then, of course, the Ben Johnson thing exploded. But my father got me Winstrol™ for my Christmas stocking. My father is a school teacher. He's got a master's degree, and he's an athlete. He's a smart guy, but he didn't know what steroids were, and nobody did in 1981. In fact, even I used to say, "My doctor said that they're vitamins for athletes." That's how I looked at them.

Dad had a prescription from a doctor, so it wasn't like I would go down to the drug dealer. My father filled it at [the] pharmacy for his son's Christmas. And he kind of said, "I don't know about these things. I know the pharmacist," he said. "Watch out for these things." I would say, "Dad, they're vitamins. I train harder than usual people." Of course, everybody knew I was a nut. So he said, "Yeah, okay." He just figured they were special vitamins.

Author: And the media?

Frattasio: Of course, as the media educated people, we know differently now. Everybody knows. But then it was no big deal. Everybody knew I was taking steroids. I've seen that change over the years as people have become educated. It was secretive then because people wanted you to believe that they were doing it themselves. The biggest problem with people lying and saying they're not on [steroids] is that they want credit for their gains. I personally had no problem with it because, being a strong person inside, I knew that I trained hard. I wasn't fooling myself or anybody else. I worked hard for the stuff, and I don't care what anybody thinks. A lot of people don't feel that way, and maybe they have a reason to because they're lard asses in the gym or they don't have a lot of self-confidence. But that's why people would lie.

But now, because there's such a stigma to being on drugs and taking steroids, now people really want to lie about it. They don't want to let on [that they are using them]. Steroids are really looked down on now. In the early '80s, there were entire gyms that were 'roid gyms. Now it is very hush, hush. Most owners don't want steroids in their gym because it gives the gym a bad name. They don't want parents to keep their kids from buying gym memberships because they're afraid they're going to get steroids at their gym. I used to shoot people up in the college center bathrooms with people walking in and out. And it was like, "These are 'roids, this is important."

I couldn't seeing myself doing that today. I mean, needles, syringes, drugs, and people seeing that—it's a whole different attitude. Things have changed. Society has changed its view.

Author: So society has changed in its attitude towards steroids?

Frattasio: Definitely.

Author: How?

Frattasio: The media. I always thought that the media would never do anything about steroids, but I was wrong. The media has helped. The media still puts people on steroids, but they've really helped to give steroids a black eye. They've done a good job.

Sporting events such as the 100-meter sprint are measured in such tiny units. Remember, Ben Johnson used steroids and beat Carl Lewis by only 13/100 of a second! Let's look at some of the real cost of using steroids. Ben Johnson had a promising career ahead of him. Even if he had not been caught, he would have the gold medal unfairly. No one knows how much money he would have earned as the world's fastest man. Here are a few of the problems that Ben has had to face since the '88 Summer Olympic games:

September 1988	Wins the gold medal.
September 1988	Three days later, tested positive for steroids; his medal is taken away.[2]
October 1988	Charged with pointing a starter's pistol at a driver.[3]
January 1989	Is banned from competing for two years.[4]
March 1989	His coach said that he had used steroids since 1981.[5]
May 1989	Gets into a fight with five men.[6]
April 1990	Is sued by his agent for $425,000.[7]
November 1991	Found guilty of hurting a former track teammate.[8]
January 1993	Tested positive for steroids at indoor meet in Montreal.[9]
March 1993	Is banned from competing in track events for life.

Steroids Are Cheating

Let's face the facts. Using steroids, or any other artificial method to improve performance, is cheating—plain and simple. Some athletes use them because they want to have that extra advantage over their opponents. Others say that they have to use steroids just to keep up.

But society can have an effect on steroid use. It already has. Steroid use is no longer as open as it used to be. Sure, some athletes still use them. Professional athletes, the ones who earn huge contracts based on their performance, will probably continue to use them. But the real impact that society can have is to prevent young people from using them. Their young bodies have not yet grown up, and the steroids can do much more harm. Attitudes, especially those of the father of the fifteen-year-old boy described above, have to change. They have to change in order to protect our young from hurting themselves with something that they do not fully understand.

What Can We Do?

What can society do to help the cause even further? Dr. Charles Yesalis of Pennsylvania State University suggests four ways to fight the problem.[10] First, more money should be used to put steroid pushers in jail. We have to get the big distributors, because if only the smaller ones are busted, then others will just take their place.

The second tactic is education. Educating students and teachers on the effects of steroids has helped a great deal, but more is needed. As long as there are people out there who want to use steroids, there will be people who want to make money selling them. It is a simple law of supply and demand. If you cut the demand, then the supply will decrease.

The third tactic for beating steroid use is to conduct random, unannounced urine tests in high school. It is important that these tests are not advertised. This tactic worked pretty well at the 1987 Zurich World Class track and field meet. More than half of the twenty-eight athletes scheduled for the shot put, javelin, hammer, and discus events did not show up once they heard that there would be urine testing for drugs. If a young person will not listen to the medical dangers of steroid use, then let him or her take the chance of being caught and suspended from playing sports. The fear of being kicked off the team appears to be greater than the fear of getting bad side effects. However, the adolescent who is using steroids just to look good is not affected by threats of disqualification.

More testing has other problems. Each of these tests can cost up to $200 each. Many schools cannot afford that expense. In addition, there are laws that protect people from having their private lives invaded.

The last tactic is to change our focus on winning. It is too bad that the values of sports are bigger, taller, stronger, and faster. These are very tough items to change. Perhaps it should start in the peewee baseball, football, and hockey leagues. It is surprising to see the amount of pressure that is put on these kids. Children imitate those around them. If they have a coach that screams at them to win at all costs, then they will grow up with values that are likely to invite steroid use.

Questions For Discussion

1. Do you think that there are drugs that professional basketball and football players could take that would make them perfect as jockeys in horse racing? If there were such a drug, would it be fair for them to take it?

2. How would you feel if a classmate beat you in a contest for the best short story but you later found out that he or she took a drug that made him or her write better?

3. How do you think steroid use is affected by peer pressure?

4. What kinds of things can you and your classmates do to reduce steroid use in your school?

10
Getting Help

One of the most difficult things you might have to do is to tell a friend that they have a drug problem and need help. You might even think that it is better to ignore the problem and it will go away by itself. Sometimes, you might be afraid that the person with the problem will get angry with you for pointing out his or her drug problem. If this person is in your group of friends, you might be afraid that the rest of the group will not like you. Having read Chapters One through Nine of this book, you know that a young person can be hurt by steroids.

Tell-Tale Signs of Steroid Use

The first step is to become familiar with the signs of steroid use. Steroids can cause many changes in a person. However, since most users are very secretive about their use, they may try to hide the fact that they are taking them. There are four types of changes that can occur.[1] The first change is social. This includes changes in the ways in which the person interacts with other people. The second type of change is physical. This includes changes to the person's body. The third type of change is behavioral. This includes more severe changes in how the person acts with other people. The fourth type can only be measured by a doctor. These are the changes in the person's body chemistry, which are found by testing their blood and urine. It is important to remember that a person is not necessarily a steroid abuser if he or she has a few these signs. The profile, or type, and number of signs is the most important factor.

One of the early signs of steroid use is a change in friends. All of a sudden, the person is hanging out with a new group. He or she may have recently joined a health club or a gym. If these friends are very well built and other physical signs exist, then it is possible that your friend is using steroids. Another sign is that your friend may become overly interested in health, exercise, and even weight lifting. They may take large amounts of vitamins and eat meals with many calories.

The physical signs may be easier to see, especially if you spend a lot of time with this person. For example, a rapid gain in weight and an increase in muscular development are the first signs of steroid use. In particular, steroids make the shoulders and neighboring muscle groups disproportionately large compared to the rest of the body. So a user's body looks slightly "out of proportion." Stretch marks on the skin covering chest muscles, near the attachment points on the shoulder, are another sign of steroid use because the drugs cause the chest muscles to grow faster than the skin can stretch above them.

Physical Changes That Can Occur in Steroid Abusers:

Male:
✓ Larger Breasts
✓ Smaller Testicles
✓ Lower Sperm Count

Female:
✓ Deeper Voice
✓ More Body Hair
✓ More Facial Hair
✓ Smaller Breasts
✓ Menstrual Irregularities

Both Males and Females:
✓ Acne
✓ Hair Loss
✓ Mood Swings
✓ Upset Stomach
✓ Rapid Weight Gain
✓ Difficulty in Urinating

In women, body hair may increase, and the voice may get deeper. Steroids often increase the number of pimples on the face and back. The hair on the top of the head may become thin, and the person's feet and hands may become puffy. This is because water stays in the body longer. These are changes that you, as a good friend, might notice.

The behavioral changes can be very subtle. However, they can also be very dangerous. The person may become hyperactive and more irritable. You might notice this when there is a conflict. The person on steroids may be more likely to lose his or her cool and yell at you. They can become more aggressive. Many times this occurs during athletic competition, but more and more cases happen off the playing field. Perhaps the most common time is in a car. Steroid users may lose their patience and yell at other drivers, assault them, or run them off the road. The most severe form of steroid abuse can lead to behaviors that are like some psychiatric diseases. If a person thinks about killing himself or herself, then this is the time to act. A person is crying out for help when they talk about suicide.

Finally, certain laboratory tests can tell if a person is using steroids. Finding traces of the steroid in the person's urine is the most convincing test. But sometimes the abuser stops taking the steroids a few weeks before the appointment with the doctor. Then it is likely that all of the steroid will have been removed from the urine. Doctors can now measure the amounts of testosterone and its first breakdown product, epitestosterone. But the body reacts to the steroids differently; some organs may be more affected than others. Certain hormones that are released from the brain are decreased. Liver function is changed, so the amount of various liver enzymes increases. This means that the liver cells have been damaged.

If you are using steroids, then you should give a copy of this book to a good friend of yours. Because when you begin to have problems, you will be the last to admit it. You will probably want to continue taking them. You will have to count on your friend to notice the changes in you. Hopefully, he or she will have the courage to help you.

Drug-Free Sports

Many athletic groups are making it easier to compete without having to take drugs. The number of drug-free bodybuilding and weight lifting competitions is increasing. In order to compete, you must be clean for a year. Some of the organizations even use lie detector tests to be sure.

There are many alternatives to using steroids and other drugs in order to improve performance. Sometimes a change in the training schedule and the location will help eliminate boredom. In fact, many athletes begin to look seriously at steroids when they lose their energy and their training is not going well. They are looking for motivation.

One of many alternative training procedures is called The Zero Effort Principle. This training technique was developed by Scott Chinery.[2] Chinery claims that the most important factor in increasing muscle size is the intensity of the workout. This is how hard you work over a short period of time. The basic idea of this technique is that you lift a weight as much as you can until your muscles become so tired that they will not move any more. Then you have your training partner help you lift the weights, but you must lower them on your own. You continue until you

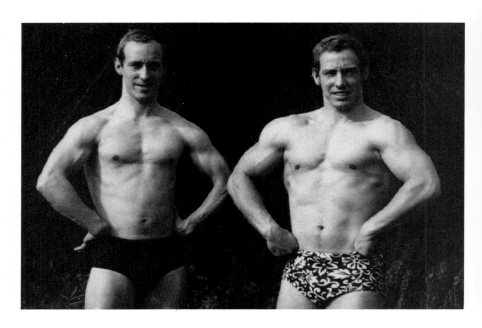

A photograph of identical twin brothers, Otto and Ewald Spitz of Germany, displays different physical characteristics based on the type of exercise in which they specialize. Otto (on the left) is a runner while Ewald is a weight lifter. This is a good example of how genetics and environment, such as exercise, can make a very big difference in physical appearance.

can no longer move the weight up or down. You must quickly switch to the next exercise since the beneficial effects of the training are lost if the muscles are allowed to rest. Chinery has seen major improvements with this method of training.

Go the Natural Route

Many very successful baseball, basketball, and hockey players have made it to the top without steroids. When they are asked what the most important factors for improving performance are, they say: proper training technique, hard work and practice, good eating habits, proper rest, and a good attitude about yourself.

If you decide that you are going to be on the Olympic team next year in a sport that you just started two days ago, be prepared for disappointment. You must learn to be patient. Set many, but smaller, goals that you can actually meet. Keep a log book of your training so you can measure your progress. The occasional victory over each of the goals can be a real boost for your morale and that's a good reason to celebrate.

Questions For Discussion

1. Why do you think the physical signs of steroid use are different in males and females?

2. How can peer pressure be used to get someone off steroids?

3. What is meant by the "natural route" of success.

Notes by Chapter

Introduction

1. J.M. Schrof, "Pumped Up," *U.S. News and World Report,* 112 (1992), pp. 54-63.

2. M.H. Williams, *Beyond Training: How Athletes Enhance Performance Legally and Illegally* (Champaign, IL.: Leisure Press, 1989).

Chapter 1

1. S.J. Winters, "Androgens: Endocrine Physiology and Pharmacology," *NIDA Research Monograph Series 102* (1990), pp. 113-130.

2. R.G. Hoskins, *Endocrinology; the Glands and Their Functions* (New York, NY.: W.W. Norton, 1941)

3. A.A. Berthold "Transplantation de Hoden," Archives of Anatomical Phsysiology, *Wisconsin Journal of Medicine,* 16 (1849), pp. 42-46.

4. C.R. Moore, *Sex and Internal Secretions,* ed. E. Allen, C. H. Danforth, and E. A. Doisy (Baltimore, MD.: Williams & Wilkins, 1939), pp. 354-451.

5. E.C. Brown-Sequard, "The Effects Produced in Man by Subcutaneous Injection of a Liquid Obtained from the Testicles of Animals," *Lancet,* 2 (1889) pp. 105-107.

6. C.D. Kochakian, "History of Anabolic-Androgenic Steroids," *NIDA Research Monograph Series 102* (1990), pp. 29-59.

7. A. Butenandt, "Ueber die chemische Untersuchung der Sexualhormon," *Z. Angew. Chem.,* 44 (1931), pp. 905-908.

8. K. David, "Uber des Testosteron, des Kristallisierte Mannliche Hormon aus Steerentestes," *Acta Brev. Neerland Physiol. Pharmacol. Microbiol.* 5 (1935) pp. 85-86.

Chapter 2

1. E. Marshall, "The Drug of Champions," *Science,* 242 (1988), pp. 183-184.

2. M. S. Bahrke, C. E. Yesalis 3rd, and J. E. Wright, "Psychological and Behavioral Effects of Endogenous Testosterone Levels and Anabolic-Androgenic Steroids among Males," *Sports Medicine 10* (1990), pp. 303-337.

3. C. E. Yesalis, "Epidemiology and Patterns of Anabolic-Androgenic Steroid Use," *Psychiatry Annual,* vol. 22, 1992, pp. 7-18.

4. B. Gilbert, "Drugs in Sports," *Sports Illustrated 30* (June 30, 1969), pp. 30-42.

5. C. E. Yesalis, R. T. Herrick, W. E. Buckley, K. E. Friedl, D. Brannon, et al., "Self-Reported Use of Anabolic Androgenic Steroids by Elite Powerlifters," *Physician & Sportsmedicine,* 16 (1988), pp. 91-100.

6. W. A. Anderson, M. A. Albrecht, D. B. McKeag, D. O. Hough, and C. A. McGrew, "A National Survey of Alcohol and Drug Use by College Athletes," *Physician & Sportsmedicine,* 19 (1991), pp. 91-104.

7. L. N. Burkett, and M. T. Falduto, "Steroid Use by Athletes in a Metropolitan Area," *Physician & Sportsmedicine,* 12 (1984), pp. 69-74.

8. W. E. Buckley, C. E. Yesalis, K. E. Friedl, W. A. Anderson, A. L. Streit, J. E. Wright, "Estimated Pevalence of Anabolic steroid Use among Male High School Seniors," *Journal of the American Medical Association,* 260 (1988), pp. 3441-3445.

9. J. C. Cohen, T. D. Noakes, and A. J. Spinnler Benade, "Hypercholesterolemia in Male Power Lifters Using Anabolic Androgenic Steroids," *Physician & Sportsmedicine,* 16 (1988) pp. 49-56.

10. H. G. Pope Jr., D. L. Katz, and R. Champoux, "Anabolic-Androgenic Steroid Use among 1,010 College Men," *Physician & Sportsmedicine,* 16 (1988) pp. 75-81.

11. M. H. Williams, "Beyond Training: How Athletes Enhance Performance Legally and Illegally," (Champaign, IL.: Leisure Press, 1989).

12. R. Johnson, *Monitoring the Future: A Continuing Study of the Lifestyles and Values of Youth* (Ann Arbor, MI.: University of Michigan Institute for Social Resources, 1990.)

13. J. Ross, F. Winters, K. Hartmann, et al., *1988-89 Survey of Substance Abuse Among Maryland Adolescents* (Baltimore, MD.: Maryland Department of Health and Mental Hygiene, Alcohol and Drug Abuse Administration, 1989).

14. R. H DuRant, V. I. Rickert, C. S. Ashworth, C. Newman, and G. Slavens, "Use of Multiple Drugs Among Adolescents Who Use Anabolic Steroids," *New England Journal of Medicine*, 328 (1993), pp. 922-926.

15. Vince Stigler, personal communication, (July, 1993).

16. T. Dezelsky, J. Toohey, R. Shaw, "Nonmedical Drug Use Behavior at Five United States Universities: A 15-Year Study," Bulletin on Narcotics, 27 (1985), pp. 45-53.

Chapter 3

1. W. O. Johnson, and K. Moore "The Loser," *Sports Illustrated*, 69 (1988) pp. 20-27.

2. R. Voy "Drugs, Sports and Politics," (Champaign, IL.: Leisure Press, 1990).

3. D. Catlin, R. Krammerer, C. Hatton, M. Sekera, and J. Merdink, "Analytical Chemistry at the Games of the XXIIIrd Olympiad in Los Angeles, 1984," *Clinical Chemistry*, 33 (1987) pp. 319-327.

4. E. Marshall, "The Drug of Champions," *Science*, 242 (1988) pp. 183-184.

5. C. E. Yesalis, W. A. Anderson, W. E. Buckley, and J. E. Wright, "Incidence of the Nonmedical Use of Anabolic-Androgenic Steroids," *NIDA Research Monograph Series*, 102 (1990), pp. 97-111.

Chapter 4

1. J. D. Wilson, "Androgens," *The Pharmacological Basis of Therapeutics*, ed. A. G. Gilman, T. W. Rall, A. Nies, and P. P. Taylor (New York, NY.: Pergamon Press, 1990).

2. A. J. Ryan, "Anabolic Steroids Are Fool's Gold," *Federal Proclamation*, 1981, pp. 2682-2688.

3 .D. L. J. Freed, A. J. Banks, D. Longson, and D. M. Burley, "Anabolic Steroids in Athletes: Crossover Double-Blind Trial on Weightlifters," *British Medical Journal*, 2 (1975), pp. 471-473.

4. E. Marshall, "The Drug of Champions," *Science*, 242 (1988), pp. 183-184.

5. J. A. Lombardo, "Anabolic-Androgenic Steroids, in Anabolic Steroid Abuse, ed. G. C. Lin and L. Erinoff, *NIDA Research Monograph Series*, 102 (1990), pp. 60-73.

Chapter 5

1. H. A. Haupt and G. D. Rovere, "Anabolic Steroids: A Review of the Literature," *American Journal of Sports Medicine*, 12 (1984), pp. 469-484.

2. R. H. Strauss, and C. E. Yesalis, "Anabolic Steroids in the Athlete," *Annual Review of Medicine*, 42 (1991), pp. 449-457.

3. J. M. Schrof, "Pumped Up," *U.S. News and World Report*, vol. 112, 1992, pp. 54-63.

4. O. Fultz, "Roid Rage," *American Health*, 10 (1991), pp. 60-65.

5. A. J. Ryan, "Anabolic Steroids Are Fool's Gold," *Federation Proceedings* 40 (1981), pp. 2682-2688.

6. K. E. Friedl, "Reappraisal of the Health Risks Associated With the Use of High Doses of Oral and Injectable Androgenic Steroids," *NIDA Research Monograph Series*, 102 (1990), pp. 142-176.

7. Ibid.

8. R. Goldman, *Death in the Locker Room: Steroids and Sports*, (South Bend, IN.: Icarus Press, 1984).

9. H. Sklarek, R. Mantovani, and E. Erens, "AIDS in a Bodybuilder Using Anabolioc Steroids," *New England Journal of Medicine*, 311 (1984), p. 1701.

10. Fulz, pp. 2682-2688.

11. Goldman.

12. Fulz, pp. 60–65.

13. Sklarek, Mantovani, and Erens, p. 1701.

Chapter 6

1. J. P. Freiner and W. Alvarez, "Androgen-Induced Hypomania," *Journal of Clinical Psychiatry*, 46 (1985), pp. 354-355.

2. H. G. Pope and D. L. Katz, "Affective and Psychotic Symptoms Associated with Anabolic Steroid Use," *American Journal of Psychiatry*, 145 (1988), pp. 487-490.

3. W. R. Annitto, and W.A. Layman, "Anabolic Steroids and Acute Schizophrenic Episode," *Journal of Clinical Psychiatry*, 41 (1980), pp. 143-144.

4. H. G. Pope and D. L. Katz, "Bodybuilders' Psychosis," *Lancet*, 1, (1987), p. 863.

5. T. P. Su, M. Pagliaro, P. J. Schmidt, D. Pickar, O. Wolkowitz, and D. R. Rubinow, "Neuropsychiatric Effects of Anabolic Steroids in Male Normal Volunteers," *Journal of the American Medical Association*, 269 (1993), pp. 2760-2764.

6. R. H. Strauss, J. E. Wright, G. A. M. Finerman, et al., "Side Effects of Anabolic Steroids in Weight-Trained Men," *Physician & Sportsmedicine*, 11 (1983), pp. 87-96.

7. R. H. Strauss, M. T. Ligget, and R. R. Lanese, "Anabolic Steroid Use and Perceived Effects in Ten Weight-Trained Women Athletes," *Journal of the American Medical Association*, 253 (1985), pp. 2871-2873.

8. H. A. Haupt, and G. D. Rovere, "Anabolic Steroids: A Review of the Literature," *American Journal of Sports Medicine*, 12 (1984), pp. 469-484.

9. H. G. Pope, and D. L. Katz, "Homicide and Near-Homicide by Anabolic Steroid Users," *Journal of Clinical Psychiatry*, 51 (1990), pp. 28-31.

10. T. Chaiklin and R. Telander, "The Nightmare of Steroids," *Sports Illustrated*, 69 (1988), pp. 82-102.

11. G. N. Conacher, and D. G. Workman, "Violent Crime Possibly Associated with Anabolic Steroid Use," *American Journal of Psychiatry*, 146 (1989), p. 679.

12. B. Jancin, "Is Athlete's Steroid Use a Valid Insanity Defense?," *Clinical Psychiatry News*, 17 (1989), pp. 2-15.

13. R. T. Rada, D. R. Laws, and R. Kellner, "Plasma Testosterone Levels in Rapists," *Psychosomatic Medicine*, 38 (1976), pp. 257-268.

14. H. B. Moss, G. L. Panzak, and R. E. Tarter, "Sexual Functioning of Male Anabolic Steroid Abusers," *Archives of Sexual Behavior*, 22 (1993), pp. 1-12.

15. Ibid.

Chapter 7

1. J. V. Brady, and S. E. Lukas, *Testing Drugs for Dependence Potential and Abuse Liability* (Washington, DC.: U.S. Superintendent of Documents, 1984).

2. C. E. Yesalis, J. R. Vicary, W. E. Buckley, A. L. Streit, D. L. Katz, and J. E. Wright, "Indications of Psychological Dependence Among Anabolic-Androgenic Steroid Abusers," ed. G. C. Lin and L. Erinoff,

Anabolic Steroid Abuse, Washington, DC: U.S. Superintendent of Documents, *NIDA Research Monograph Series,* 102, (1990), pp. 196-214.

3. S. E. Lukas, "Current Perspectives on Anabolic Androgenic Steroid Abuse," *Trends in Pharmacological Science,* 14 (1993), pp. 61-68.

4. G. Ariel and W. Saville, "Anabolic Steroids: The Physiological Effects of Placebos," *Medicine and Science in Sports,* 4 (1972), p. 124.

5. K. J. Brower, G. A. Eliopulos, F. C. Blow, D. H. Catlin, and T. P. Beresford, "Evidence for Physical and Psychological Dependence on Anabolic Androgenic Steroids in Eight Weight Lifters," *American Journal of Psychiatry,* 147 (1990), pp. 510-512.

6. K. J. Brower, "Addictive Potential of Anabolic Steroids," *Psychiatric Annals,* 22 (1992), pp. 30-34.

7. K. J. Brower, F. C. Blow, J. P. Young, and E. M Hill, "Symptoms and Correlates of Anabolic-Androgenic Steroid Dependence," *British Journal of Addictions,* 86 (1991), pp. 759-768.

8. F. Tennant, D. Black, and R. Voy, "Anabolic Steroid Dependency with Opioid-Type Features," *New England Journal of Medicine,* 319 (1988), p. 578.

9. K. B. Kashkin, and H. D. Kleber, "Hooked on Hormones? An Anabolic Steroid Addiction Hypothesis," *Journal of the American Medical Association,* 262 (1989), pp. 3166-3170.

10. K. J. Brower, "Clinical Assessment and Treatment of Anabolic Steroid Users," *Psychiatric Annals,* 22 (1992), pp. 35-40.

11. Ibid.

Chapter 8

1. Adam Frattasio interview with author, Belmont, MA (July 1993).

2. A. Frattasio, "Full Circle on Steroids," *Muscular Development,* (August 1993), pp. 128-130.

3. Ibid.

Chapter 9

1. Adam Frattasio, interview with author, Belmont, MA, (July 1993).

2. D. Benjamin, "Shame of the Games," *Time,* 132 (October 10, 1988), pp. 74-77.

3. "Johnson Charged in Pistol Incident," *Jet,* 75 (October 31, 1988), p. 46.

4. R. O'Brien, "Ben Again," *Sports Illustrated*, 78 (March 15, 1993), p. 9.

5. M. Noden, "A Dirty Coach Comes Clean," *Sports Illustrated*, 70 (March 13, 1989), pp. 22-23.

6. "Ben Johnson Gets into Scuffle with Five Men," *Jet*, 76 (May 29, 1989), p. 50.

7. "Sprinter Johnson Sued by his Canadian Agent," *Jet*, 77 (April 2, 1990), p. 46.

8. "Ben Johnson Guilty in Teammate Assault," *Jet*, 81 (November 11, 1991), p. 47.

9. "Ben Johnson is Barred for Life from Track and Field After Testing Positive for Steroids," *The New York Times*, March 6, 1993, p. 32.

10. C. Yesalis, "Steroid Use Is Not Just an Adult Problem," *The New York Times*, December 4, 1988, p. 12.

Chapter 10

1. W. A. Narducci, J. C Wagner, T. P. Hendrickson, and T. P. Jeffrey, "Anabolic Steroids—A Review of the Clinical Toxicology and Diagnostic Screening," *Journal of Toxicology and Clinical Toxicology*, 28 (1990), pp. 287-310.

2. S. Chinery, *Anabolic Steroids and Bodybuilding* (Toms River, NJ.: SMS Publishing, 1983), pp. 81-84.

Index

stanozolol, 24, 29
sterility, 66
Stigler, Vince, 18
strength, 39
strychnine, 4
syringes, 90
tennis players, 19
testes, 35
thyroid hormone, 35
tobacco cigarettes, 18
toxic effects, 44, 47-51
track and field, 19
tumors, 61

U

urine testing, 24, 29, 93

V

violent behavior, 56, 62
vitamins, 89, 96

W

weight lifters, 15, 39, 56, 99
Winstrol, 73, 75, 76
withdrawal, 59, 68, 70

Y

"Year of Steroids", 17
Yesalis, Dr. Charles, 92

Z

Zero Effort Principle, 99, 101